COORDINATING COMMUNITY SERVICES FOR THE ELDERLY

COORDINATING COMMUNITY SERVICES FOR THE ELDERLY

THE TRIAGE EXPERIENCE

Joan Quinn, R.N., M.S.
Joan Segal, M.A.
Helen Raisz, M.A.
Christine Johnson, R.N., M.S.

Editors

Foreword by Congressman Claude Pepper

SPRINGER PUBLISHING COMPANY
New York

Springer Publishing Company, Inc.
200 Park Avenue South
New York, New York 10003

82 83 84 85 / 10 9 8 7 6 5 4 3 2 1

Library of Congress Cataloging in Publication Data

Main entry under title:

Coordinating community services for the elderly.

  Bibliography: p.
  Includes index.
  1. Community health services for the aged.
2. Community health services for the aged—
Connecticut. 3. Triage, Inc. I. Quinn, Joan.
RA564.8.C654   362.1'9897'009746   81-18407
ISBN 0-8261-3300-2   AACR2
ISBN 0-8261-3301-0 (pbk.)

Printed in the United States of America

Contents

Foreword

Medicare was enacted by Congress in 1965 to provide a federally sponsored health insurance program for persons over 65 and persons eligible for Social Security disability benefits. The design of this program was to provide a reimbursement mechanism for this population that would ensure payment for basic medical care required to treat acute, short-term health problems. The Medicare program represented a commitment of this nation's resources to guarantee that no older adult would go without basic medical care. An important assumption in the development and enactment of this legislation was that a major impediment to gaining access to basic health services was the inability to pay for such care.

Over the past 15 years it has become evident that assured reimbursement does not necessarily guarantee access to appropriate care. The nature of this nation's health care delivery system has been both shaped and limited by the public and private reimbursement policies permitting payment for health care. The hearings conducted by the House Select and Senate Special Committees on Aging have shown that home care services which can reduce or prevent the need for institutional care are less likely to receive reimbursement than institutional care itself, even though the former may be more appropriate to an individual's needs.

Elderly persons in this country should not have to endure the difficulties which they encounter under our current health care system to receive adequate and appropriate health services. The Triage project is one of several federally sponsored research and demonstration programs designed to develop a better way to provide health care to the older American. The success experienced by Triage is worthy of consideration by persons throughout this nation who want to make our health care system better. It is the belief of many of us in Congress that individual communities and organizations can take the initiative to implement those positive aspects of innovative health care programs such as Triage. We believe that the information contained in this book will be helpful to that end. We commend the contents of this book to your attention in the hope that each town and municipality throughout this nation will actively and energetically work to provide better, more appropriate health care alternatives for this country's elderly citizens.

                              Claude Pepper
                              Chairman, Select Committee on Aging
                              U. S. House of Representatives

Preface
The Word "Triage"

The word "triage" is attributed to Napoleon who, during the European war of 1804, used it to describe the process by which decisions were made about attending the wounded. Napoleon advised dividing the wounded into three groups: those who were going to die no matter how much attention they received; those who were going to recover even without immediate attention; and those who, without immediate attention, would die or be severely disabled (the most critical group). The word is now used in much the same way in Mobile Army Surgical Hospitals (M.A.S.H.), in hospital emergency rooms, and at disaster scenes.

The meaning of the word as used by the Triage project is entirely different. The project does not "triage" people by grouping them according to who can be expected to live and who can be expected to die. Rather, going to the roots of the French language before Napoleon's coinage, the Triage project uses the word in the sense of the verb *trier*, which means to pick, to sort, to choose. What Triage does is to choose from among a wide range of services those which will make the greatest difference in mitigating or compensating for functional dependency and those which will enhance the quality of life of the older adult.

Editors and Contributors

Joan Quinn, *R.N.*, *M.S.*, is Executive Director of Triage, Inc., and Executive Director, Management Staff of Connecticut Community Care, Inc. A frequent lecturer at local, state, and national meetings, Ms. Quinn has also authored several articles and participated as panelist in numerous programs. In addition, she has presented testimony before the U.S. Senate Finance Committee and the Special Committee on Aging, the U.S. House of Representatives Select Committee on Aging, and the National Commission on Social Security. Ms. Quinn is a member of many professional organizations and committees, and has served on several task forces. Among her most recent honors was her selection as representative to the 1981 White House Conference on Aging. Over the past several years she has held faculty appointments in the departments of Social Work, Nursing, and at the Health Center of the University of Connecticut, as well as at the Universities of Hartford and Bridgeport. She holds B.S.N. and M.S. degrees from the University of Connecticut and is a certified geriatric nurse practitioner.

Joan Segal, *M.A.*, Research Associate at Triage, Inc., was a Research Associate at the University of Connecticut School of Dental Medicine, Department of Behavioral Sciences and Community Health before joining the Triage staff. Ms. Segal was an editor of *Triage: Coordinated Delivery of Services to the Elderly* and had major editorial responsibility for *Group Practice and the Future of Dental Care*, edited by C. R.

Jerge, et al. She presented a paper at the 57th General Session of the International Association of Dental Research, New Orleans in 1979 and has co-authored several articles. She is presently completing a Master of Science degree in Community Health from the University of Connecticut.

Helen Raisz, M.A., is a Research Associate at Triage, Inc. Ms. Raisz is currently working on a Ph.D. in Sociology from the State University of New York at Buffalo. Her research interests include gerontology, interorganizational relations, and social theory. She has presented papers at the Gerontological Society's 30th Annual Scientific Meeting and the American Public Health Association Annual Meetings in 1976 and 1979. She has also contributed to several other papers and presentations. Ms. Raisz was an editor of *Triage: Coordinated Delivery of Services to the Elderly*, 1979. Prior to joining Triage, she was a Research Associate at the University of Connecticut Health Center.

Christine M. Johnson, R.N., M.S., is presently Assistant Director, Medical Nursing at Hartford Hospital, Hartford, Connecticut. Prior to this position, Ms. Johnson was a nurse-clinician at Triage, Inc. for three years. Her professional activities include membership on the board of directors of the Connecticut Nurses' Association and the American Heart Association of Greater Hartford. Ms. Johnson holds a nursing diploma from Hartford Hospital, a B.S. degree from Central Connecticut State College, and an M.S. in Medical-Surgical Nursing from the University of Connecticut.

Edgar Bernier, M.B.A., is Claims Manager, Assistant Fiscal Officer of Triage, Inc., responsible for all provider claims and reimbursement functions, and for management of all service provider contracts. Mr. Bernier is a member of several honor societies, and he also serves on the State Advisory Committee on Home Health Care, Regulations and Certificate of Need. He received his master's degree in Health Care Administration from the Bernard M. Baruch College in New York.

Joseph Hodgson, M.S.W., is Assistant Director, Community Relations at Triage, Inc., where his functions include compilation of research statistics, government and provider relations, and individual case management. In addition, he maintains an independent private practice of individual, marital, and family psychotherapy. Mr. Hodgson has served on a variety of professional committees and is frequently a lecturer and consultant on aging. He is a graduate of Trinity College and the University of Connecticut Graduate School of Social Work.

David Rieck, M.B.A., Associate Director of Triage, Inc., has been responsible for the finance, personnel, purchasing, and administrative functions at Triage, including development of cost retrieval and grant preparation for funding sources, since 1974. He has also served as consultant to local nursing home facilities. Mr Rieck is a member of several health care associations. He holds a Connecticut Nursing Home Administrator's License, a B.B.A. degree in Management, Marketing, and General Business from Western Michigan University and an M.B.A. from the University of Hartford.

Nancy Ryan, R.N., M.S., is Assistant Director, Clinical Services at Triage, Inc. Ms. Ryan holds American Nursing Association certification as a geriatric nurse practitioner and an advanced nursing administrator. In addition, Ms. Ryan has faculty appointments to the University of Connecticut School of Nursing and Central Connecticut State College. She is a frequent lecturer and has served on numerous professional committees and task forces. Her recent publications include articles in the *AORN Journal* and the *Journal for Gerontological Nursing*.

Acknowledgments

We gratefully acknowledge the many Triage staff members who provided us with their valuable input throughout the preparation of this book. Special thanks go to Debbie Oakes, who patiently and always with good humor typed and retyped the innumerable drafts of our manuscript.

We are also indebted to the members, both past and present, of our Triage Board of Directors, who volunteered their time and efforts to ensure the continuing success of our project. Their sense of commitment to Triage and to the elderly people we serve has been unfailing over the past seven years.

These acknowledgments would not be complete without mentioning the motivating force behind our efforts—the elderly clients themselves. In our endeavors, we have considered the clients our partners. The client-centered approach that is the heart of the Triage process could not have succeeded without their commitment to and enthusiastic support of the project.

Our gratitude extends to the National Center for Health Services Research, Office of the Assistant Secretary for Health, Department of Health and Human Services, which supported the research between April 1, 1976, and March 31, 1979 (Grant Number HSO2563); to the

Connecticut State Department on Aging, which supported project operations from 1976 to 1979; and to the Health Care Financing Administration, Department of Health and Human Services, which has provided continued funding under Grant Number 95–P–97371/1–01.

1

Introduction: The Need for a Client-Centered System of Long-Term Care

JOAN QUINN, R.N., M.S.

> Care of the frail elderly may be our most wicked problem in human services . . . as with other wicked problems, there is not a consensual problem definition. Is the problem too much care or too little care? Is the problem professional indifference toward the aged? Changing family values? Excessive attempts to prolong life? We have heard all these diagnoses and more, but there is no agreement. (Taber, 1980)

Over a decade ago, social scientists, policy makers, and care planners articulated the major dilemma encountered in providing long-term care for the elderly and disabled: how to attain the goals of quality of care and cost containment at the same time. Today, this dilemma has become compounded by the larger numbers of older persons who are living 20 to 30 years beyong retirement at age 65. Despite the rapid growth of America's elderly population, there has been no large-scale development of a system of medical and social services capable of meeting the needs of this population.

Current Dilemmas in Long-Term Care

As in the past, physical and mental disabilities are today the most dreaded hazards of growing old. At the same time, changing social currents are affecting the impact of these disabilities on the individual, the family, and society. A noted gerontologist, the late Margaret

1

Blenkner, outlined three ways to cope with what she and others have termed the normal dependencies of aging: the self-solution, the kinship solution, and the societal solution (Blenkner, 1969). Retirement or the loss of a supporter or companion leaves many elderly people with inadequate financial and emotional resources for the self-solution to be viable. Turning from an inadequate self-solution to the kinship solution, they may find that, because of the mobility of this society, children are less likely to live with or near their aging parents than was true in the past. Moreover, in families where both husband and wife work, there is less time—and perhaps less inclination—to provide for elderly and often ailing parents (Kamerman, 1976). Despite these factors, care of the elderly and disabled by families is widespread (Shanas et al., 1968; Congressional Budget Office, 1977), yet, excessive burden on the family is often given as the primary reason for seeking admission to a long-term care facility (Litman, 1971). The inability of many families to cope adequately with the problems of aging has put more and more pressure on the societal solution to supplement, but not supplant, the self- and kinship solutions.

Society is, at present, ill-equipped to respond to the challenge of providing long-term care in a comprehensive manner. More often than not public resources for delivering care outside of an institution are inadequate. Eligibility requirements for publicly-funded home or community-based services are categorical and restrictive. Often those benefits that are received are too little, too late.

The emphasis of the contemporary long-term care system is clearly on institutional facilities. This institutional bias restricts the use of home health and other alternative services that often would be more appropriate in meeting the varied needs of the elderly. While medical care to the acutely ill is often individualized according to specific need, personal care delivered over time to the chronically ill is not. Cousins (1979) has stated somewhat ironically that the hospital is the worst place to be for someone who is critically ill. One might legitimately ask whether nursing homes are the most appropriate placement for most people in need of long-term personal care.

Yet, even with the undue emphasis on nursing homes and other institutions, the financing mechanism for institutional care is inadequate. To become eligible for Medicare (Title XVIII) reimbursement, one must meet strict definitions of medical necessity related to diagnosis; to become eligible for Medicaid (Title XIX), one must meet equally strict definitions of medical indigency. Unable or unwilling to meet these eligibility requirements, many elderly people sick enough to be considered for placement in long-term care institutions are receiving little or no regular medical care (Williams, 1973).

The even greater problems the elderly face in attaining long-term care outside the walls of a nursing home have been summarized succinctly by the National Academy of Sciences (1977):

> Pluralism and specialization in the delivery of services often mean that elderly individuals are forced to seek the assistance of several providers or programs in order to obtain a necessary complement of services. Limitations in functional capacity, confusion engendered by differences in eligibility requirements for services, and limitations in the scope of services offered by some programs make the arrangement of a care program very difficult for many elderly individuals . . . .

A disintegrated system for providing home-based services is aggravated by an abundance of inadequate financing mechanisms.

Initiation of a systems approach to address the problems of organizing and financing long-term care is further thwarted by three decision-making processes at work in the existing health care network. They include the decision making of service providers, third-party public and private reimbursement systems, and elderly people and their families. These three processes mutually reinforce each other, with each actor in the system making decisions based on perceptions of how the other actors will respond, rather than on perceptions of client need.

Providers decide which services to render based almost entirely on fiscal considerations. For example, although the professional leaders in the field, represented by the National League for Nursing, have identified 23 home health services as essential for the well-being of older persons, the majority of visiting nurse associations can afford to offer only the six services that are reimbursable under Medicare guidelines. Similarly, third-party payers look to the providers to decide what amount to pay for a service based on guidelines set by the providers as to what constitutes a reasonable and customary charge or allowable cost. Given the decisions already made by providers and payers, the client is forced to choose not the service most appropriate for his or her needs, but only that service offered by the provider and reimbursed by the third-party payer. For example, a client who is no longer able to shop for food or prepare meals might choose to have "meals on wheels" delivered to the home. Because this is a minimally reimbursable service, few home-delivered meal services have been developed in the community, with the result that the client may be forced to choose nursing home placement merely to meet his or her nutritional needs.

The Alternatives Concept

While the dilemmas of long-term care are far from resolved, the official policy of the U.S. government has clearly moved in the direction of establishing health care programs that will correct the institutional bias and remove many of the organizational and financial barriers to a comprehensive, coordinated continuum of care for the elderly at the community level (Doherty, Segal, and Hicks, 1978). Over the past decade, the Department of Health and Human Services has departed from a services strategy, which emphasized providing additional services such as day care and homemaker service (Weiler, 1978), to a systems strategy based on a channeling agency concept.* Several small-scale research and demonstration projects have been mounted. Georgia Alternative Health Services, Monroe County Community Long-Term Care, Wisconsin Coordinated Care for the Elderly, Washington Community-Based Care for the Functionally Disabled, Minnesota Healthy Seniors Center, New York Long-Term Home Health Care, and On Lok Community Care for Dependent Adults are among the most notable of these (Galblum, 1980).

Project Triage, one of the oldest and most sophisticated of the demonstrations, was ahead of its time. In 1977, when the National Academy made its recommendation that "a single agency should be identified to coordinate the delivery of health and social services to the dependent elderly at the community level," Triage had been doing precisely that for three years. To overcome the current state of fragmentation and other organizational problems, Triage developed a new system which linked personal care, medical care, income maint-

*"The term 'channeling' refers to the organizational structures and operating systems required in a community to link people who need long-term care to the appropriate services. At the core of channeling are client assessment and case management as methods for organizing care to meet individual needs and controlling long-term expenditures" (DHEW, 1980).

enance, and family support. The system was designed to assess client needs; integrate the provision of appropriate medical, mental health, and social services; and monitor their quantity and quality. Individual choice of in-home, community, and institutional services to meet documented need was the primary consideration in the development of this alternative system. To overcome the current financial barriers, Triage devised an uncomplicated reimbursement system, providing single-entry to a billing system as well as single-entry to a services system. This removed much of the web and the weight of the current paperwork associated with paying for the care of the chronically ill.

In sum, the objective of Triage was to develop a system which offers enough choice so that, subject to reasonable financial constraints, services can be prescribed that are appropriate to an individual elderly person's needs. Unlike the traditional system, in which the services provided to an individual depend upon what is available and reimbursable, Triage organizes available services around the needs of the client, develops new services when needed ones are not available, and assures that all needed services are adequately monitored and reimbursed. In other words, rather than bending the client to meet the requirements of the system, the system is adapted to meet the individual needs of the client.

Policy Concerns

When the concept of an alternative, single-entry assessment, coordination, monitoring, and reimbursement system was first discussed, many concerns were raised. First was the fear that the cost of such a system might be prohibitive—that total health care costs might be significantly higher. This fear proved unfounded. The process of assessment, coordination, and monitoring has been shown to pay for itself by containing total expenditures for health care, and by substituting, when appropriate, community and in-home services for institutional services.

The second concern was that the provision of home care services would have an add-on effect. Comprehensive home care services are not considered to be part of the continuum of medically necessary services and, therefore, have never been significantly reimbursed. At the present time, home health expenditures account for less than 2 percent of the total expenditures of Medicare and Medicaid (Fisher, 1980). Hitherto unavailable to society, with certain exceptions, home services have not developed beyond the level of inspirational volunteerism. Home care and community-based service providers find themselves in a dilemma. They recognize their need to move from volunteerism to professionalism but realize that this may mean relinquishing their claim to be cheaper than an institution. While home care services are usually a less expensive substitute for institutional services, this may not continue to be so as home health providers become more professionalized and regulated. Triage has demonstrated that in many cases, home and ambulatory services can indeed substitute for institutional services, but the result is not always a corresponding reduction in total health expenditures. However, because home services are a substitute for institutional services, there generally is no add-on effect.

A third concern of policy makers was that a system such as Triage would have a case-finding effect. In other words, elderly persons not currently known to the existing system might be drawn into the alternative care system. Again this was not the case. Older adults have usually entered the care system if they have had problems. Where they entered the system, and whether this access has resulted in resolution of their problems, are questions that must be answered.

Over the past five years, Triage has addressed these concerns and proven itself to be a straightforward system that works. A client-centered, comprehensive health care system has developed that can ensure utilization of services appropriate to client need, while retaining effective control over the costs of care.

Policy Implications

The current structure of the health care system for elderly persons is such that the determination of appropriate care is made primarily by those persons who provide services. However, specific service providers often have only fragmentary knowledge of the comprehensive needs of the older adult, the type of alternative services available, and the costs of services rendered. To say that the solution to this dilemma is to improve the knowledge and expertise of service providers in these three areas is only partially correct. Improving the knowledge of both consumer and provider is important. However, to expect that the professional service provider will acquire additional skill and responsibility outside of his/her area of expertise may be unreasonable; it will do little to improve the effectiveness of the health delivery system. The focus of the health care professional ought not be diverted from improving the skill with which he/she delivers the health care service itself. Nor will escalating health care costs be effectively controlled by having third-party payers constrain the amount and types of services eligible for reimbursement in a manner unrelated to consumer needs. Such a practice merely results in a shift to services which are reimbursable. The problems of high cost and excessive rates continue uncontrolled.

The concept of a comprehensive assessment, coordination, and monitoring function performed by an organization comprised of interdisciplinary, expert professional teams is not new. What is new is the direct connection of this function to the control of reimbursement. It is the integration of these two tasks—coordinating care and controlling costs—at the local or regional level, that has the potential for improving the effectiveness and efficiency of the current health care system. The results that have been observed in central Connecticut are that local community and regional resources can be mobilized to complement existing services to provide adequate care, without necessarily generating a host of new professional services. Triage has demonstrated that it is possible to provide the comprehensive array of medical and social services necessary to minimize the amount of deterioration in functioning status which accompanies advancing age. Further, it has shown that this full spectrum of services can be provided at a cost which does not have to be significantly higher than that which a comparable group of older persons would expend for fewer services delivered in a haphazard fashion.

The succeeding chapters describe in detail the development and implementation of the Triage model of a client-centered system of community long-term care. Chapter 2 focuses on the mechanics of implementing the Triage concept, the problems encountered, and the strategies required to undertake a similar project. The chapter concludes with an overview of the unique features of the model as it emerged during its mature, operational phase. The funding of services and operations is documented with historical illustrations. Chapter 3 describes the development, coordination, and reimbursement of the full spectrum of services required to meet the medical and social needs of the elderly. The use of the assessment process to develop a comprehensive data base from a holistic health perspective is described in Chapter 4. Chapter 5 describes the process that assures that the right service is delivered at the right time in the right manner in terms of both quantity and quality. The findings which resulted from the research designed to assess the ability of Triage to meet its goals are summarized in Chapter 6. This research effort included a longitudinal study that examined changes in functioning status and patterns of service utilization and expenditures for the entire Triage population. Chapter 7 suggests administrative and legislative initiatives for replicating the Triage model in other localities.

The lessons provided through the development and testing of the Triage model suggest a direction which offers hope to policy makers, providers, and elderly consumers for a system more efficient and responsive than the currently existing system.

2

A Client-Centered Care System: From Idea to Implementation

HELEN RAISZ, M.A. AND DAVID RIECK, M.B.A.

The Triage model project began operations on February 1, 1974, but its historical roots go back at least as far as the 1971 White House Conference on Aging. Studies prepared for that conference indicated that on both the state and federal levels, health services for the elderly were far from ideal.

Generalized concern over the deficiencies was soon translated into four specific goals:

1. To serve the growing number of elderly people in need of health and supportive services;
2. To contain the steadily increasing costs of health and supportive services;
3. To demonstrate the effectiveness of alternatives to institutionalization for elderly persons in need of long-term care;
4. In sum, to develop an alternative public policy to solve the complex problems of long-term care, consistent with the public's ability and willingness to pay for humane and effective care.

To achieve these goals, programs were proposed that would expand the spectrum of services available to the elderly, coordinate these services, and experiment with varying methods of reimbursement. It was believed that such programs would shift the emphasis from

9

frustrating, episodic, inpatient treatment to long-term, integrated support outside the walls of an institution.

At the federal level, interest in these programs was translated into enabling legislation through the passage of Section 222(b) of PL 92-603, the Social Security Amendments of 1972. Concurrently, at the state level, other activities were undertaken as part of the necessary preparation for the joint venture in federal-state cooperation which came to be known as the Triage project. These activities are described in the following section.

Initial Planning

Inspired by the platform of the White House Conference on Aging, the Executive Secretary of the Connecticut Commission on Aging addressed a short letter to the governor:

> May I present an idea for your consideration? I would propose that the state develop a plan which would provide guaranteed social security for the many neglected, isolated, and lonely elderly in our state . . . . It is my conviction that this could launch an original, humanitarian, pioneering effort by our state towards meeting the complex needs of our elderly citizens. (Bloom, 1971)

The governor was receptive to the idea and suggested the formation of a task force to study the feasibility of a home care program for the elderly. The efforts of this task force were well received, and resulted in a request from the governor that the Commission on Aging undertake an in-depth study of home care.

The Home Care Study Committee produced a work plan outlining seven major tasks:

1. Assess the extent of need for home care among Connecticut's elderly;
2. Ascertain the extent of home care services presently available;
3. Design a questionnaire for local visiting nurses associations to provide data and evaluations to the Home Care Committee;
4. Prepare a legislative proposal to help close the gap between the needs assessed and the services presently available;

5. Identify the sources of funding by program and governmental level (local, state, or federal);
6. Identify choices which would have to be made about establishing a program in terms of: (a) type of service, (b) geographic coverage, (c) organization;
7. Establish a three-year program for phasing in a personal care system.

In addition to outlining these tasks, the committee established five guiding principles for the proposed organization:

1. Coordination, possibly through regionalization, is needed to make the delivery of services more efficient.
2. Arrangements should be made which would "minimize the financial activity of participants in the program"; in other words, the program should cover, as does Medicare, even the "undeserving rich."
3. Whatever the sponsoring organization, there should be a meaningful policy voice from senior citizens.
4. The organization should emphasize outputs, the actual satisfaction of the needs of the clients, rather than the inputs of particular programs.
5. Flexibility is a most important characteristic to be kept in mind at all times.

Fundamental to these principles was the logic of Dr. Ian R. Lawson, the experienced geriatrician on the Home Care Study Committee who stated:

> If the ill effects of aging can be defined as the loss of options in life, care of the elderly can be defined as a systematized attempt to recover or find alternatives to some of these lost options . . . .
> With limited funds available, the strategy of spending should recognize that ten dollars spent higher up on the spectrum of care will achieve very little; spent lower down, it may make a significant difference in the life of the elderly person. (Lawson, 1975)

Dr. Lawson developed "A Check List for Community Planning of Resources for the Elderly," in which he suggested that a successful program must include three elements:

1. *A variety of services: the personal need for a spectrum of services.*
   Elderly people do not have single, stereotyped needs, whether
   these needs be for types of accommodation or for recreation.
   For example, if a community has ample nursing home beds but
   lacks special residential apartments or other alternatives to
   institutionalization, elderly people may be placed in circum-
   stances of unreasonable dependency which is both dehuman-
   izing and wasteful.
2. *True complementarity of agency workings: the operational need
   for a spectrum of services.* No single agency could possibly
   embrace the hugely varied and complex needs of the elderly.
   Many disciplines are involved through a number of agencies.
   Nevertheless, the community can reasonably expect evidence
   of inter-agency cooperation; that is, integrated planning of
   agency development, cooperation at the casework level, and an
   absence of wasteful, competitive duplication.
3. *Good case coordination, with sensitive, flexible professionals.*
   Case coordination should individualize the situation of persons
   being served, provide continuity and comprehensiveness, and
   involve other agencies in a harmonious way. Only fully prepared professionals have the knowledge, skills, and attitudes
   required to perform effective case coordination.

The Search for Funding

After one year of concentrated work by the committee, the Home Care
Report was accepted by the governor. An underlying philosophy, a
conceptual model, and a commitment concerning care for the elderly
were embodied in the master plan. The next task was to seek funding to
create an organization which would realize the goals inherent in the
planning design. A discrepancy soon arose between planning aspir-
ations and the resources necessary to translate the dream into reality.
While the need for a wide variety of services was abundantly clear, the
planning staff faced the possibility that, despite some minor but
propitious changes in the Medicare law, progress would be limited by
funding restrictions.

Several funding sources, both public and private, were explored.

The possibilities included federal funding under Title III (Model Projects) of the Older Americans Act, Titles VI (Social Services), XVIII (Medicare), and XIX (Medicaid) of the Social Security Act, and the Model Cities Program, and private funding from the larger local corporations. After all of these possibilities were examined closely, five funding sources were identified as promising: The Federal Administration on Aging, the Health Services Administration, Medicare, Medicaid, and private insurance vendors. A request to one of these sources, the former Health Services Administration, fell on responsive ears. An official of that organization suggested that the Triage model might possibly be funded as a research and development project by the National Center for Health Services Research under Section 222 of Public Law 92-603.

The decision to seek federal funding for Triage as a research and development project, rather than as a service model, necessitated a linkage with an institution of higher education which would have the requisite research capability. The University of Connecticut Health Center was chosen to provide that linkage.

Prior to grant application, the Home Care Committee prepared a table of organization, an outline of the flow of services, and an evaluation of possible service regions. However, as work progressed on the application, it became evident that the actuarial expertise of those working on the grant was insufficient. This was an important consideration since the creation of an appropriate fiscal system would be vital to the success of Triage. A meeting with representatives of the insurance industry and the State Insurance Department was arranged to discuss fiscal policy. As a result, Triage, from the outset, was guided by sound insurance principles.

In compliance with the grant procedure established in the state, letters of support were sought from the state agencies (the Department of Health and the Department of Finance and Control) and the community organizations (planning agencies, hospitals, visiting nurse agencies) that might lend endorsement and assistance to the Triage project. These letters were, on the whole, favorable and enthusiastic, and were included in the grant proposal.

Concurrent with the preparation of the application, the state legislature moved to create the Connecticut Council on Human Services. This council was designed to integrate the policy and funding of eight separate state departments (Social Services, Health, Mental

Health, Mental Retardation, Education, Children and Youth Services, Aging, and Community Affairs). The Council on Human Services was legislatively empowered to develop no fewer than two pilot demonstration projects. The Council viewed Triage as a model transferable to other age groups and to other human services, and as a means of strengthening the capacity of the state to facilitate human service delivery. In late 1973, Triage became a priority project of the Council.

A consortium of already existing non-profit agencies and consumers, rather than a new single agency, was proposed to govern the project through contract with the Department on Aging. Until the consortium became a legal entity, a well-established home health agency in the region agreed to be the "lead agency" or sponsor for the project. The Council on Human Services served in an advisory capacity.

Three years after the commissioner's initial letter, the cornerstones for the Triage project had been laid. The vision of the original planners, the hard work of the Home Care Committee, the persistence of the director of the Council on Human Services in keeping the idea alive, her success in securing start-up funding, and the cooperation of the "lead agency" all served as decisive influences in the implementation of this project. The pioneering effort of the state of Connecticut toward meeting the complex needs of its elderly citizens was ready to commence.

As formalized in the grant application to the National Center of Health Services Research, the objectives of the Triage project were to:

1. Provide a single entry mechanism to coordinate the delivery of institutional, ambulatory, and in-home services on behalf of the elderly client;
2. Develop necessary preventive and supportive services;
3. Develop an integrated service delivery system at the local level;
4. Obtain public and private financial support for the full spectrum of services;
5. Demonstrate the cost-effectiveness of coordinated care, including care to prevent illness, compensate for disability, and support independent living at home; and care prescribed appropriate to need rather than according to third-party payer service restrictions.

Setting

The area chosen in which to develop and test the model was the seven-town Central Connecticut Planning Region (see Figure 2–1). This region, which includes rural, urban, and suburban areas, was selected after consultation with potential consumers, as well as with a wide array of providers and governmental agencies. In the proportion of the elderly among the total population, their ethnicity, and socioeconomic factors, the Central Connecticut Region was fairly typical of the rest of the state and the nation. Thus, it was deemed a suitable microcosm in which to test the Triage model.

Initial Operations

Triage assessed the first client on March 1, 1974. In the previous months, the Home Care Committee had confronted and solved the problem of selecting a suitable person to administer this complex system. In the final blueprint of the project, the broadly based skills and training of a nurse-clinician were considered crucial to the proper functioning of the Triage design. Such skills and training included a firm background in clinical assessment techniques, an understanding of the relationship of social and psychological factors to the total health and independent functioning of an elderly person, and a broad knowledge of the community and its supportive agencies. A nurse-clinician with these qualifications was chosen as director of the Triage project.

Three principal challenges faced the new director and her advisors. The recruitment, orientation, and training of an interdisciplinary team of health professionals that reflected the staffing design was a primary concern. Another immediate need was the establishment of a board of directors. If Triage was to conform to its stated goals and objectives, it was essential that it be acknowledged as an autonomous legal entity. The third major challenge was to achieve stable funding. These three challenges had to be addressed simultaneously.

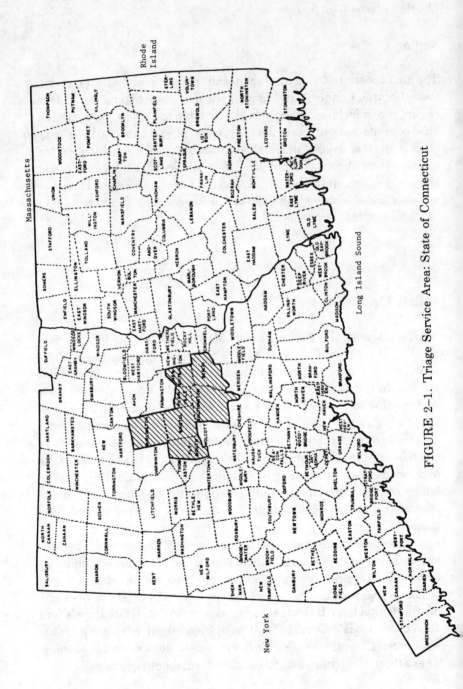

FIGURE 2-1. Triage Service Area: State of Connecticut

Staffing

During the initial operational phase, considerable effort went into the recruitment of staff. The director maintained scrupulously high standards in assessing the clinical and administrative skills of qualified professionals. The care taken in hiring personnel proved to be important because Triage derived much of its strength and direction from the concentrated expertise of its core staff. The first people hired served as role models for those who followed.

The efforts of Triage to provide a comprehensive assessment of its elderly clients, and to coordinate, monitor, and reimburse a wide range of services, required a multidisciplinary staff with intimate knowledge of the service and reimbursement systems. To manage a single-entry system of medical and social service delivery, clinical staff members were required to have education and experience in either nursing or social work. To manage a single-entry reimbursement system, administratrive staff members had to have a background in business administration, accounting, data processing, and secretarial science. The staffing pattern is sketched in Figure 2–2.

Recruitment and hiring of staff were carried out incrementally as the caseload grew. The first person hired by the executive director was the business manager. In addition to assisting the executive director and managing the business side of the enterprise, the business manager developed accounting and data processing procedures. The second person hired was a caseworker who, together with the executive director (acting as the nurse-clinician), formed the first interdisciplinary team.

Development of the Clinical Staff. As the news about the organization spread by word of mouth, the number of referrals made by elderly individuals or their advocates grew, necessitating that two nurse-clinicians and two caseworkers be added to the clinical staff. During 1975 and the beginning of 1976, two more interdisciplinary nurse-caseworker teams joined the staff. By April of 1976, the Triage clinical staff had grown to ten, comprising five clinical teams. Two more clinical teams were added over the next two years.

Whenever an interdisciplinary approach is undertaken, role tension between disciplines is inevitable, and the new Triage organization did not escape this problem. Professionals trained in different disci-

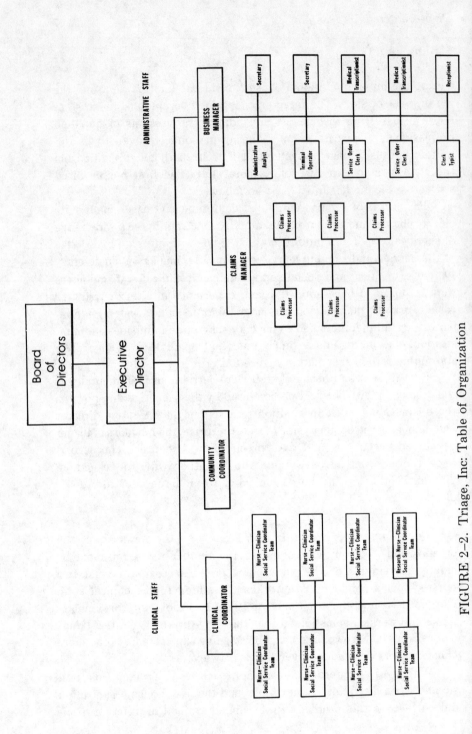

FIGURE 2–2. Triage, Inc: Table of Organization

18

plines are not accustomed to working together in an intensive way. Moreover, their backgrounds give them differences in orientation and expectation. Social workers tend to be more concerned with process, while nurses are more action oriented. A balance has to be achieved if the greatest benefit for the client is to be attained. As the Triage organization evolved, the roles within it were evolving, too. Role conflict was to be expected and welcomed as an opportunity to question, to analyze, to resolve, and to improve.

Role tension between the nurse-clinicians and the caseworkers developed as a result of several factors. When Triage began in 1974, medical services (such as physicians, hospitals, visiting nurses, and home health aides) were relatively available. In contrast, few social services were directed toward the needs of the elderly. Consequently, the caseworkers, who were ideally to be coordinators of social services, found little to coordinate. Instead, they provided direct casework services, advising the clients. Since there were no social agencies to turn to, if the caseworkers felt a client needed a service such as mental health counseling, they provided it themselves. The result was that the caseworkers, hired as members of assessment and referral teams, found themselves bogged down with casework and separated from the main Triage process.

A second contributing factor to the role conflict resulted from the lack of role models for the caseworkers. The nurse-clinicians could look up to the executive director as a leader in their field, but because the community coordinator position was not filled for many months at a time, there was no representative of the social work profession to serve as a mentor.

The third factor creating role tension was the overlap of functions that each member of the team expected to perform. This was exacerbated by the differences in educational level in the early days of the project. Generally, the nurse-clinicians had higher academic credentials; most of them held master's degrees, while most of the caseworkers were on the bachelor's level. Through their academic training and clinical experience, these clinicians had acquired a sophisticated understanding of social service problems and felt capable of performing many functions that were traditionally within the domain of the social work profession. Nurse-clinicians had extensive coursework in gerontology, as well as considerable clinical experience with the elderly. In contrast, most of the caseworkers were recent graduates and lacked experience.

A fourth factor was the way that the teams were to operate. From the beginning, it was the caseworker's job to monitor clients who had been assessed by the nurse-clinician to insure that services were provided as prescribed and that they continued to be appropriate to the client's needs. The caseworker also reported changes in the client's status to the nurse-clinician. However, the nurse-clinician went out alone to perform assessments of the individual clients. Although the caseworker was trained in psychosocial assessment and aware of the medical problems of the elderly, the only part of the assessment he/she completed was the financial section, in which a client's assets and expenditures were evaluated and eligibility for programs was determined.

The caseworkers were dissatisfied not only because the nurse-clinicians were performing some functions that they felt they themselves should be doing, but also because they felt separated from the assessment process. This separation denied them the opportunity to express their opinions regarding a client's condition and kept them from the first-hand, baseline knowledge of the client that they needed in their discussions with the nurse-clinicians.

In response to the caseworkers' grievances, as well as to the work demands involved in handling a growing caseload, it became logical for the nurse-clinicians to share more of the assessment burden with the caseworkers. As a reflection of the added responsibility and accountability assumed by the social workers, their job title was changed from caseworker to social service coordinator. From that time on, the social service coordinator and the nurse-clinician generally performed as a team in the initial assessment of clients who were referred to Triage. This arrangement resulted in greater job satisfaction for the social worker and better shared knowledge of the client's needs. To keep this new joint team functioning at a skilled professional level, Triage upgraded the prerequisites for the position of social service coordinator. The new requirements for both practical experience and the acquisition of a master of social work degree (MSW) made the social worker's position more comparable to that of the nurse-clinician.

Not all of the Triage staff were comfortable with the shifting nature of their responsibilities. There were those who did not feel secure in a position that often required autonomous judgment concerning a particular course of action. Although the social service coordinators and the nurse-clinicians were only supposed to provide client assessment, coordination, and monitoring of services, sometimes, in an emergency, they found it necessary to intervene. There were those on the staff who did not like the responsibility of having to make sudden decisions. Some would have been happier in a work situation where their roles would be more clearly defined and their responsibilities more clearly delineated.

The caseload was set arbitrarily at 250 clients per team or 125 clients per clinical staff member. This caseload was found to be too high for those teams with high risk, unstable clients. Because clients were referred sequentially, it was impossible to know in advance how many clients a team could handle. For clients with less involved problems it would, of course, take less time to assess and to arrange for services. Those high-risk clients with multiple problems would take more time, as would those clients who, though better off physically, might be lacking family support and be in danger of institutionalization. As frustrating as too high a caseload migh be, too low a caseload could prove just as detrimental. The cost for such a caseload would be unrealistic and would not conform to public policies or be acceptable to government agencies. The goal of 250 clients per team was kept in order to be as cost-efficient as possible, but the teams transferred clients among themselves in order to maintain a balance between high and low risk clients.

Because of the growth of the clinical staff, the problem with role conflict, and the increase in the complexity of the organization, the executive director found it necessary to delegate some of her supervisory duties to a clinical coordinator. The nurse-clinician who held this position was responsible for overall service delivery, public relations, and educational activities, as well as for carrying a caseload. As administrative duties grew, the clinical coordinator played an increasingly important role in professional staff development. She organized in-service programs for both Triage staff and contracted providers, directed the orientation of new staff members, and supervised a quality assurance program.

Administrative Staff. Like the clinical staff, the Triage business staff grew as the number of client referrals grew. The greater number of clients brought a greater need for administrative functions, as well as an ever increasing stream of paperwork. It became necessary to supplement the early administrative staff of business manager and clerk-typist by creating new administrative positions. One of these positions was executive secretary to the executive director. Another was that of administrative analyst, whose functions included managing the claims transmittal file, the payroll, and accounts payable, and reporting claims statistics. A medical transcriptionist who typed client records was also hired, as was a switchboard operator-receptionist who took referrals, directed clients to the proper department, and facilitated inter-departmental communication, as well as communication between Triage and the public.

On the higher administrative level, an assistant business manager joined Triage early in 1975. He originally shared responsibilities with the project's business manager. However, in November of 1975, the institution of a Medicare waiver system, in which customary reimbursement limitations were removed, brought much greater Triage involvement in fiscal matters and brought the assistant business manager much greater responsibility.

With the granting of waivers, the Triage project began to deal directly with the Division of Direct Reimbursement (DDR), the government fiscal intermediary.* This made it necessary for Triage to set up a claims operation. The assistant business manager was responsible for developing and supervising this huge claims function. Under the procedures made possible by the establishment of this new department, providers would submit their bills directly to Triage, whose staff would check the validity of all charges. Triage, in turn, would submit all acceptable charges to the Division of Direct Reimbursement for payment.

This process necessitated two kinds of personnel. At one end of the process were service order clerks who typed service orders as dictated by the nurse-clinician/social service coordinator teams. At the other end of the process were the claims processors who checked whether the services documented in provider bills were identical to those authorized in the service orders.

In addition to their paperwork, the claims processors had personal contact with Triage clients. Clients, when they called about a claim,

---

*The Division of Direct Reimbursement is now the Office of Direct Reimbursement, Social Security Administration, Health Care Financing Adminstration.

would ask by name for their own claims person. The claims personnel came to know some of the clients rather well. Through such personal involvement, business staff members saw themselves not as fillers of faceless forms, but as essential links in the chain of care that provided services to "Mr. Smith" or "Mrs. Jones."

As in other areas of the Triage operation, personnel to fill these positions were hired only as they were needed. Two clerks were able to handle the volume of service orders. However, more people were required to process the provider claims which were sent to the Triage office daily. The number of claims processors varied according to the number of claims to be processed, although it was determined that six people were sufficient to process effectively the number of claims generated by the Triage providers.

Teamwork. The staffing pattern of Triage was characterized by teamwork at two levels. At the level of client contact, nurses and social workers worked in consort. At the agency level, clinical and administrative staff worked cooperatively.

The stratification that usually exists in a large organization was broken down by the fact that both the administrative staff and the clinical staff recognized an interrelatedness of purpose. They understood that one area could not be separated from another. Every job was necessary and important. No job could be done in isolation. Besides exercising skills in a particular area of expertise, each staff member understood the function of every other member of the organization. This interdependence and equality, coupled with the complete understanding each staff member had gained of his/her own role, led to the mutual respect, cooperation, and efficiency that characterized the Triage staff, enabling it to meet the project's goals.

The Triage Board of Directors

At the same time that the internal structure of Triage was being built, another evolutionary, incremental process was taking place: establishment of a board of directors that would serve to sanction Triage as an autonomous legal entity. Over a 16-month period, the governing body of Triage evolved through four stages:

1. An advisory committee,
2. An advisory board,
3. A policy board, and
4. A full-fledged board of directors for the free-standing corporation, Triage, Inc.

Each succeeding stage represented the assumption of greater commitment and responsibility for the affairs of the Triage project.

Much of the groundwork for securing suitable community representation on a governing board was undertaken during the beginning months of Triage operation. At this time, preliminary interviews were held with the directors of health and social service agencies within the seven-town region to seek their cooperation with the new organization. Some initial reservations were expressed by service agency directors, but gradually Triage staff developed strong working relationships with the community agencies. The inter-agency communications that were established served as a foundation for the formation of the consortium of providers and consumers that eventually was to govern Triage.

Early in 1974, an advisory committee was formed for Triage's sponsor or "lead agency," a local home health agency. This advisory committee was comprised of Triage staff members and representatives from the State Council on Human Services, the State Commission on Aging, and various community agencies. The committee met for two months and addressed many issues pertaining to the formation of a board of directors. These issues concerned size, sphere of responsibility, and composition of the proposed board. After giving much consideration to determining an optimal balance between lay and professional membership, the advisory committee felt reluctant to resolve the issues addressed. Such policy decisions were left for the advisory board that evolved from the advisory committee.

The advisory board was composed of many of the representatives that had been serving for the initial two-month interval. In addition to Triage staff and agency representatives, members of the elderly population from the seven-town region were included on the advisory board. The inclusion of consumers was a critical feature of the Triage governing board. As consumer representatives became familiar with serving in this advisory capacity, they proved to be important advocates for Triage in the region. As a group, they constituted the most stable element on the advisory board.

After meeting for two months, the advisory board determined that when the board of directors was formed, the board should assume the authority to ensure compliance with its decisions. As a step toward this end, the advisory board changed its title to that of policy board.

In June of 1974, a charter was prepared by selected members of the policy board and presented to the entire board for consideration. At this juncture, the representatives of the provider agencies expressed an unwillingness to act. They hesitated to make legal commitments for their agencies. As a consequence of the uncertainty that prevailed among provider members, a task force of five representatives from the total policy board prepared a "memo of understanding." The memo was designed to make necessary revisions and additions to the charter. Legal commitment from the agencies that signed the memo of understanding was no longer required, but the acknowledgment of their willingness to work toward the development of a legal entity was directly implied.

The policy board met monthly from December 1974 through June 1975 to prepare for the transition from a board which was merely advisory to a board which would be a governing body, bearing full responsibility for the property and affairs of an autonomous corporate entity. During this time, issues such as the nomination and election of directors and the adoption of bylaws were resolved. On June 2, 1975, a certificate of incorporation for Triage, Inc. was filed with the secretary of state.*

The charter members of the board of directors included 11 provider members, one member each from the boards of the four local hospitals and seven community health agencies. Seven consumer representatives, defined as persons 60 years of age or older, one from each of the towns in the region, also served on the board. Later, representatives of the medical societies and the community mental health center were invited to join as additional provider members.

Throughout the four evolutionary stages of the board of directors,

---

*The purposes of the corporation as stated in Article II of the bylaws are: "to make provisions for services within the Central Connecticut Planning Region; to coordinate the activities of other agencies in providing such services; to gather information and to conduct studies with respect to the conditions of elderly persons and their need for particular services and appropriate means of satisfying such needs; to receive funds from federal, state, municipal, and private sources; and to apply such funds for the purposes herein before stated."

the executive director maintained a pivotal position and exerted a strong guiding influence. She sought cooperative, positive action from the board and often met personally with individual board members to foster constructive interaction. As long as Triage, Inc. operated under the guidelines of the state and federal grants, the scope of governance of the board was limited to "housekeeping matters," communication, and long-range planning. The executive director made most of the decisions concerning program goals, personnel, and clientele. The board of directors, especially the officers serving as the executive committee, provided her with strong support.

Through the phases of advisory committee, advisory board, policy board, and finally board of directors, consumer and provider representatives worked together to guide, advise, and govern the activities and policies of Triage. The board was exemplary in putting the good of the region ahead of the particular interests of any one town or provider. Although its sphere of governance was restricted by federal and state guidelines, within its defined scope the board functioned efficiently and industriously. Board members were committed to the goals of the project and received personal satisfaction in contributing to such an ambitious undertaking—an undertaking that offered the potential to make an important impact on the lives of the elderly in their region and in the nation.

Stable Funding

Funding is fundamental. Without stable funding, the staff, no matter how qualified, cannot meet the needs of its clients, and the board of directors, no matter how willing to take responsibility, will have nothing to govern. Therefore, the third challenge of the organization, that of securing stable funding, was perhaps the most important. Without enough funding to allow a fledgling organization to evolve through the planning and initial operational stages, no innovative program can demonstrate the potential of the model.

While the proposal for funding the complex research and demonstration project was still being prepared, Triage began operations. At that time, the project was assured only five months of funding.

From its inception, Triage was dependent on both the State of Connecticut and the federal government for funds. During the initial five-month period, the State Council on Human Services, by assessing each of the eight separate state departments that comprised the Council, contributed $45,000 of "seed" money. In addition, the federal Administration on Aging, responding to a request from the State Council, agreed to provide $135,000. After this initial period, the State of Connecticut provided continuing funding for the daily operation of Triage, and the National Center for Health Services Research (NCHSR) funded the project's research component. The Health Care Financing Administration funded the waivered services provided to clients under the terms of the NCHSR grant.

Sustaining funding over a five-year period (1974–1979) from both state and federal sources was problematic. Funds from the National Center for Health Services Research were contingent upon approval of a proposal which had to be submitted annually by Triage and the University of Connecticut Health Center to a study section for peer review. Funds from the Council on Human Services (and later the Department on Aging) were contingent upon approval of the governor's budget submitted annually to the state legislature for political review. Triage had to fight for its fiscal survival on two fronts, state and federal, four times between 1975 and 1978, but each time emerged stronger with a new set of alliances to back its efforts the next year.

To maximize the effect of the available funds, Triage requested and received extensions on many of the early grants. The practice of conserving funds whenever possible and spreading them over a longer time period enabled Triage to remain fiscally stable.

Fiscal Management. One of the reasons that Triage was able to attract state funding was that the service waivers brought to Connecticut more than $10 for each $1 the state appropriated for the operation of the program. An equally persuasive argument was the prudent fiscal management exhibited by the administrative staff.

A major fear of those who were skeptical of the Triage concept was that operating such a project would be extremely expensive. To alleviate those fears, it was necessary to analyze the operational costs of the project. The total budget for Triage grew over 127 percent during Fiscal Years 1975–1979. Start-up costs, including costs of incorporation, establishment of accounting records, and equipment purchases, accounted for a substantial proportion of the initial costs. Concomitant with the growing number of staff positions, personnel costs grew from $14,253 in 1974 to $473,544 in Fiscal Year 1978. In terms of percentage of total costs, these figures represented an increase from 24.4 percent in 1974 to 83.1 percent in 1978. This increase paralleled the growth of the project and reflected the conservative, incremental staffing pattern of the Triage organization in which personnel were added only when an increase in the number of clients warranted it.

Triage analyzed its total budget as reflected in the five basic functions it performed on behalf of its clients. These functions were:

1. Assessment, through which initial client contact was made; all physical, social, psychological, and life support needs of the client were determined; and a plan of care was developed.
2. Reassessment, through which the client was reevaluated using a structured format; the client's needs were reappraised; and the plan of care was amended to respond to changes in the client's situation.
3. Coordination and monitoring, in which the plan of care was implemented, employing the various providers that were required to meet a client's individual needs; client and provider contact was maintained to ensure that the client's needs were being met; and service delivery was monitored for quality and quantity.
4. Claims and reimbursement, through which verification of the client's receipt of appropriate services was made and authorization for payment for services was obtained.
5. Research and development, in which data were collected for analysis to determine the effectiveness of the project.

Once total costs per month for each of the functions were determined, functional costs for each Triage client during Fiscal Year 1978, the most representative year, were calculated as follows:

1. Assessment. An average of 50 new clients per month were assessed during Fiscal Year 1978. The average cost of $100.94 per assessment is based on the $5,047 average monthly expenditures for this function (10.5 percent of total expenses).
2. Reassessment. The Triage staff completed an average of 50

reassessments per month in Fiscal Year 1978. Based on the average monthly cost of $2,917, reassessment costs averaged $58.34 per client (5.8 percent of total expenses).

3. Coordination and Monitoring. Triage served an average of 1,422 clients per month in Fiscal Year 1978. Based on the average of $21,771 spent on coordination and monitoring each month, per client costs averaged $15.31 monthly for this function (44.4 percent of total expenses).

4. Claims and Reimbursement. For Fiscal Year 1978, the Triage claims staff processed and approved an average of 4,438 claims per month. Based on an average total monthly expenditure of $13,803, Triage spent $3.11 per claim (28.5 percent of total expenses).

5. Research. An average of $5,876 per month was spent on research. However, as research was not an ongoing operational expense relating to client service, it would be inappropriate to analyze these costs on a per client basis. (Research accounted for 10.8 percent of total expenses.)

Calculated on the basis of an average caseload of 1,422 active clients per month during Fiscal Year 1978, the average monthly cost per client was $30.62, or $1.01 per client per day (see Table 2–1).

The percentage of total health expenditures that was allocated to Triage operations was 7.5 percent. This figure compares favorably with the cost of more traditional health care systems. For example, the operational costs of Part B Medicare carriers from 1967–1973 ranged from 9.7 percent to 12.4 percent of total health expenditures (U.S. Department of Health, Education, and Welfare, 1976). However, in addition to the claims review process, Triage operational costs encompassed other administrative functions not performed by the Part B carriers, including the intensive and ongoing assessment, reassessment, coordination, monitoring, and research functions. The examination of operational costs leads to the conclusion that the operational costs for a comprehensive, coordinated, community care system such as Triage are not a prohibitive factor in furthering the development of long-term care alternatives for the elderly.

TABLE 2-1. Schedule of Unit Costs FY 1978

Function	Total Cost Per Month	Percent Of Total*	Avg. Units Per Month	Cost Per Unit	Cost Per Client Year**	Cost Per Client Month**	Cost Per Client Day**
Assessment	5,047	11.5	50/mo.	100.94/ assessment	42.60	3.55	.12
Reassessment	2,917	6.6	50/mo.	58.34/ reassessment	24.60	2.05	.07
Coordination/ Monitoring	21,771	50.0	1,422/mo.	95.31/ client month	83.72	15.31	.50
Claims	13,803	32.0	4,438/mo.	3.11/ claim	116.52	9.71	.32
TOTAL	43,538	100.0	5,960		267.44	30.62	1.01

*Does not include research costs.
**1,422 Clients.

Conclusion

The implementation of an idea as complex as " a single agency to coordinate the delivery of health and social services to the dependent elderly at the community level" is a formidable challenge, the dimensions of which should not be underestimated. However, the experience of Triage has been that an incremental approach can be successful in meeting the challenges of initial acceptance and planning, staffing, governance, and funding.

The initial planning process brought together visionary individuals from both the public and private sectors and translated their global ideas into a feasible project design.

The incremental approach to staffing assured that high standards would be maintained and that only professionals with the highest qualifications would be recruited to work as partners on an interdisciplinary team.

The cautious four-stage process of moving from an advisory committee to a board of directors, with each stage reflecting increasing responsibility, resulted in the achievement of an effective governing body.

Stable funding to assure that the work of the project could continue was secured through a combination of prudent fiscal management and through exploration of a variety of funding sources at the state and federal levels.

The strong Triage organization that evolved over time is a model which potentially can be transferred to any area which sets as its goal the humane and cost effective care of the elderly.

3

Waiver Implementation, Provider Relations, and Claims Processing

EDGAR BERNIER, M.B.A.

The fragmentation which exists in the health care system for the elderly is due, in large part, to the methods of reimbursement. In this system, reimbursement is generally restricted to certain services that are specifically related to particular medical conditions, while many other needs and services are ignored. The system focuses on acute care services while neglecting services designed to prevent impairment and maintain functioning ability. The challenge facing Triage was to implement a health care delivery system for the elderly that would be based on individual need and be truly comprehensive, integrating ambulatory, home care, and institutional services to provide both acute and chronic care.

Over an initial 18-month period (February 1974–August 1975), Triage implemented a model system by bringing together the bits and pieces which characterized the "non-system" of care that already existed and developing new services to offer care alternatives. Health care was conceptualized as including both medical and social components. Triage planners concurred with Leopold and Schein's (1975) statement that "in a comprehensive approach . . . fully separated programs of medical care appear just as inconsistent and incomplete as do programs directed exclusively at social or economic needs."

August 1, 1975 was a landmark date for the fledgling project. As of that date, Triage was able to take advantage of Section 222 of the Social Security Amendments of 1972, Public Act 92-603, which, for the purposes of research, authorizes the Secretary of Health, Education, and Welfare (now Health and Human Services) to waive Medicare restrictions. This legislation permits the use of Medicare Trust Funds to create a reimbursement system which will expand coverage under the existing Medicare program and pay for many services not currently covered. The removal of Medicare restrictions enabled the elderly Triage clients to receive many needed services which, because of a lack of coverage or reimbursement, previously had been beyond their reach. The granting of the waivers was one of the most important factors in insuring the success of the project.

Waiver Implementation

The implementation of a reimbursement system is an issue of critical concern to the design of any program for the delivery of comprehensive health services. Programs that operate with public funding, in particular, are subject to serious scrutiny and weighty expectations. Reimbursement in a public program is expected to be carried out in an efficient and expeditious manner. This expectation is based on the belief that efficient processing of claims can have a positive, if indirect, effect on the population being served. Timely payment is regarded as a means of preventing provider frustration, of fostering cooperation among providers, and, ultimately, of creating community support for a program. A major challenge for the Triage project was to create a workable reimbursement system in an environment where the territory was not always charted and where the previous experience of providers had been with the complex and cumbersome machinery of the Medicare and Medicaid programs.

The cornerstone of the Triage reimbursement system was the waivers. The granting of the waivers had two major effects. First, many specific Medicare technicalities, such as benefit periods and the "skilled nursing" requirement, were waived. These technical waivers also removed several other restrictions, such as the three-day prior hospitalization requirement for nursing home care and the requirement that home care be under a physician's plan of treatment. Second, new service waivers made it possible for Triage to authorize payment for many ancillary and supportive services not traditionally covered by Medicare, such as prescription drugs, dental care, mental health services, and homemaker services.

The waivers created an entirely new coverage perspective. Wide discretionary power was given to Triage, essentially to rewrite the rules of coverage, to determine who could receive what kind of service and in what amount.

Five elements had to be addressed to create and operationalize a set of waivers to Title XVIII: coverage, reimbursement, services definition, provider eligibility, and contracts.

Coverage

Coverage refers to a predefined set of benefits and their relationship to certain conditions and prior events. For example, prior to July 1, 1981, Medicare would cover or provide benefits for skilled nursing facility (SNF) care only if a beneficiary had been in a hospital for at least three days, was transferred to the SNF within 14 days of hospital discharge, and had a "covered" or specific condition.

With the Medicare program, however, coverage ground rules are not easily deciphered. Although the *Medicare Handbook* (1979) states what services are covered under Parts A and B, the various fiscal intermediaries intepret the handbook in different ways. Thus, a person living in New Haven, Connecticut, less than 50 miles from Hartford, may find he or she is not covered for a service which would be reimbursable through the fiscal intermediary in Hartford. While most people who turn 65 assume that Medicare will take care of all their medical bills, coverage of services often falls far short of their expectations and previous experience under employment-related insurance programs. This difference between expectations and reality has been called "phantom coverage." Most older people do not realize that, generally, Medicare only pays for about 40 percent of the bills of a beneficiary (Terris et al., 1977).

Triage recognized that traditional service controls would be unnecessary and would obstruct an alternative delivery system which was to provide comprehensive services based on appropriate care and need. With authority granted for waivers to Title XVIII, the organization's next task was to identify the specific coverage limitations and exclusions which needed to be removed by the waiver mechanism.

Table 3–1 lists the technical and new service waivers that were designed to promote comprehensive service coverage for project par-

TABLE 3–1. Triage Waivers to Title XVIII (Medicare)

Technical Waivers		New Service Waivers
Waivers to Part A— Hospital Insurance	Waivers to Part B— Supplemental Medical Insurance	
1. Entitlement	1. Entitlement	1. Inclusion Part A:
2. Deductibles	2. Deductibles	a. Intermediate Care Facility Services
3. Coinsurance	3. Coinsurance	b. Residential Care Facility Services
4. Benefit Period	4. Medical Necessity	c. Day Care Services
5. Medical Necessity		d. Homemaker Services
a. Utilization Review		
b. Fourteen-day transfer requirement*		2. Inclusion Part B:
c. Three-day prior hospitalization*		a. Mental Health Counseling
d. Requirement that services be associated with a previously-diagnosed illness		b. Companion
		c. Chore
		d. Dental
6. Skilled Nursing Facility— Level of Care		e. Medical Devices—Eyeglasses, Hearing Aids, etc.
7. Home Health—Homebound Requirement		f. Medications
		g. Legal Aid
8. Home Health—Physician Plan of Care		h. Transportation
		i. Meals and Meal Delivery

*These requirements were eliminated by the Omnibus Reconciliation Act of 1980 (P.L. 96-499, Sec. 930).

ticipants. These waivers were sufficient to expand coverage so that the coordination/assessment/monitoring concept could be implemented with the necessary flexibility. A thorough discussion of the implications of each of the 39 waivers would be impossible here, but two examples should be illustrative.

An example of a technical waiver of Medicare restrictions relates to placement in a skilled nursing facility (SNF), as referred to earlier. Before July 1, 1981, a patient had to be in a hospital for three days before a stay in a skilled nursing facility would be covered by Medicare. With the waiver granted to Triage in August 1975, a patient could be admitted to a skilled nursing facility without a prior stay in an acute care setting if the placement was deemed appropriate by the Triage staff.

Companion service is an example of a new service waiver. Researchers have shown that many older people who live alone are insitutionalized prematurely, merely because they are lonely or afraid. Under a waiver that allowed Triage to provide coverage for companion service, this form of inappropriate institutionalization was avoided.

The controlling factor for Triage coverage was not the regulatory standard, which supposedly reflects a required level of illness and rehabilitative capacity; rather, it was the judgment of the project personnel who, in concert with client, family, physician, and other interested parties, arrived at the appropriate services, regardless of whether or not the client met the restrictive requirements of the regulations.

Reimbursement

Reimbursement refers to the type and amount of payment made for services deemed reimbursable under coverage provisions. While coverage provisions may limit the services eligible for reimbursement, payment limitations also discourage the types and amounts of services purchased. A physician visit may be covered; but when reimbursement is only 50 percent of the charge, such coverage is discouraging to those seeking appropriate care.

Triage was challenged to seek waivers of reimbursement limitations that were reasonable and necessary to establish the model of client-centered, cost conscious care. The integrity of the model was established by waiving the disincentives to beneficiaries that act as barriers to necessary care, while at the same time *not* waiving the disincentives to providers that act as barriers to unnecessary care. Coinsurance and deductibles were waived, while cost reimbursement and reasonable and customary charge determinations were retained. As an additional cost containment measure, Triage was successful in persuading the majority of providers to accept assignment, that is, to agree not to bill the client for any amount over and above what was determined to be the reasonable and customary charge.

Current reimbursement mechanisms were retained for services involving only technical waivers. However, new reimbursement mechanisms were required for the new services that were not included in the existing Medicare program. For those new services provided by home health agencies (i.e., homemaker, chore, and companion services), Triage adopted the cost reimbursement method, a reasonable approach in that many of the agencies delivering such services were Medicare-certified providers, already accustomed to the cost reporting mechanism. Non-certified agencies, who generally had no experience with cost reporting, received first-year technical assistance from Triage. Thus, a uniform reimbursement method was achieved for all participating home health agencies.

For other services, reimbursement methods were adopted that were familiar to the provider involved wherever possible. For services such as prescription drugs and glasses, Triage adopted the Title XIX reimbursement method, "cost plus professional fee." Dental services were reimbursed in accordance with private insurance charge screens, while taxi services were reimbursed in accordance with the method established by the Public Utilities Commission Authority.

The tailoring of reimbursement to the providers' customary operating procedures had several advantages: fees were already established, providers were familiar with the forms, and there were established procedures for reviewing rates, if necessary. Thus, introduction of an entirely new system was avoided.

Other services did not lend themselves easily to Medicare, Medicaid, or other established reimbursement formulas, and a new method had to be adopted. Independent providers of waivered new services such as chore, companion, meal preparation, meal delivery, and mental health counseling were reimbursed according to a rate negotiated between these providers and Triage. To assist the providers in the rate negotiation process, Triage developed a policy and procedures manual which describes the steps in the process of negotiating a rate for Triage covered services.

The assistant business manager had the primary responsibility for rate negotiation. When additional technical assistance was required, it was supplied by accountants from the Division of Direct Reimbursement (DDR) of the Social Security Administration in Baltimore.

Deciding on reimbursement rates was the most time-consuming aspect of the contract negotiation process, especially since there were six different bases for reimbursement—Medicare cost reimbursement formulas, Medicare reasonable and customary charges, Title XIX rate schedules, private insurance companies' charge screens, Public Utilities Commission rates, and Triage negotiated rates. Table 3–2 lists the reimbursement methods for the different types of providers.

The outcome of the reimbursement process was a system of payments that related closely to existing reimbursement procedures for comparability and ease of administration. Provider disincentives to promote unnecessary and costly services were retained, audit capability was established, and in addition, sufficient waivers of coverage and reimbursement limitations were attained to remove financial barriers to appropriate care.

Service Definition

A key feature of the waivers was to include new services which required new definitions. Where service definitions already existed in conjunction with reimbursement plans, they were adopted. Newly covered services such as prescription drugs or independent companion had to be clearly defined so that both client and provider knew what that service entailed and how reimbursement could be directly related to the tasks and functions performed.

One of the disadvantages of adopting existing service definitions is that certain activities or services may be excluded from reimbursement because they are not included in the definition. For example, existing definitions require that physical therapy services be *rehabilitative* to the client, yet, with the elderly, *maintenance* of functioning status is equally important. In designing a waiver package, one must know and understand the existing definitions of services and how they will affect the operation of the project.

TABLE 3-2. Reimbursement Methods for Triage Providers

Medicare Reasonable And Customary Charge	Medicare Cost Reimbursement	Medicaid Rate Schedule*	Private Insurance Charge Screens	Public Utilities Commission Rates	Triage Negotiated Rates
Physicians	Hospitals	Pharmacies	Dentists	Taxi Companies	Mental Health Counselors
Physical Therapists	Nursing Homes	Audiologists			Chore Workers
Medical Equipment and Supply Companies	Home Health Agencies	Hearing Aid Dealers			Companions
Laboratories	Homemaker Agencies	Optometrists			Community Service Organizations
Podiatrists	Day Care Centers	Opticians			Meals-on-Wheels
Ambulance Companies		Chaircar			

*Cost of materials plus professional fee.

Provider Eligibility

Given the coverage, reimbursement, and service definitions established through the waiver system, the next task was to define the eligibility of providers to participate. With an extension of Medicare reimbursement to such services as homemaker, chore worker, and companion, the question was raised whether those services should be delivered by Medicare-certified agencies only, or whether eligibility could be extended to other providers.

To broaden the provider base, Triage asked for and received a waiver of certification requirements. For example, proprietary agencies could participate in the experiment without licensure.* The other requirements of Medicare participation were retained to assure quality of care. Most other services were tied directly to current certification standards (e.g., pharmacies had to meet Title XIX standards). Table 3–3 presents the licensure requirements for Triage providers.

While the waiver of certification broadened the provider base, it also meant that Triage had to assume the responsibility for insuring that its providers would deliver quality care. Triage developed a quality-assurance program for such services as day care, home-delivered meals, and independent chore and companion providers. (These efforts will be further described in Chapter 5.)

Contracts

Contracts are the final element that tie together coverage, reimbursement, services, and eligibility. Contracts are necessary because the system which emerges is substantially different from the system which is superseded. Contracts serve as both the reference point and the vehicle to implement the waivers in the community. Triage established contracts with nearly 200 non-profit voluntary and profit-making institutions, agencies, businesses, and individual providers. Other providers, including approximately 360 physicians, 118 dentists, 26

---

*The Social Security Act requires that proprietary agencies be licensed in order to participate in Medicare, but the Connecticut State Department of Health only began licensing home health agencies in January of 1979. Effective July 1, 1981, the Omnibus Reconciliation Act of 1980 (P.L. 96–499) permits proprietary home health agencies to be Medicare-certified in states without home health licensure laws.

TABLE 3–3. Licensure Authority for Triage Providers

CT State Department of Health	CT State Board of Pharmacy	Public Utilities Commission Authority	Not Licensed
Hospitals	Pharmacies	Taxis	Mental Health Counselors
Nursing Homes			Homemaker Agencies
Day Care Centers			Chore Workers
Home Health Agencies*			Companions
Physical Therapists			Community Service Organizations
Medical Equipment & Supply Companies			Meals-on-Wheels
Physicians			
Laboratories			
Dentists			
Podiatrists			
Audiologists			
Hearing Aid Dealers			
Optometrists			
Ambulance/Chaircar Companies			

*Only after January 1979.

optometrists, and 25 podiatrists, delivered services to Triage clients without special contractual arrangements.

The roster of providers was remarkably stable. While each year new providers were added, some contracts were not renewed, and some providers withdrew from participation, the majority of providers (95 percent) renewed their contracts yearly. Of those who did not renew their contracts, the greatest number were in the category of independent companions. In many of these cases, Triage had merely formalized an ongoing, informal relationship that had already been established between a client and a companion. Therefore, a companion often did not choose to work for another client after the need for services by the original client no longer existed.

Provider Relations

The development and coordination of comprehensive institutional, ambulatory, and home care services would have been impossible without the cooperation of the community of providers. At the heart of every provider relationship was good will. This good will was reflected in the uniform contracts that Triage signed with all of its providers, from the largest to the smallest.

The relationship between Triage and individual providers varied with every provider group. With the hospitals, the largest, most structured of the providers, the relationship was largely *pro forma*. Triage was basically a contractual payment mechanism. It had comparatively little impact on the services that hospitals could offer. The hospitals' interactions with Triage reflected an attempt to maintain good will in the communities they were serving. Once the hospitals' concern over confidentiality of records was satisfied, Triage was able to offer them a unique opportunity for continuity of patient care.

The relationships of the visiting nurse associations with Triage had a significant impact on their programs. Because of Triage's special reimbursement mechanism, visiting nurse associations were able to contract with providers developed by Triage for the delivery of many needed but previously unavailable services, such as meals-on-wheels. Other organizations such as a community guidance clinic, whose youth became involved in the meals-on-wheels program as well as in an unofficial "foster grandparents" program, saw an opportunity to move into areas which could enlarge their scope and assist them in carrying out their agency goals.

Organizations cooperated with Triage for three reasons: they believed that Triage's efforts on behalf of the elderly were inherently right; they saw the potential benefit that Triage could bring to their own organizations; and they also considered the potential benefit that Triage could bring to the community in the creation of a cooperative spirit and in increased employment.

After the initial contracts were signed, providers became part of a team dedicated to serving the needs of each elderly client. Triage's approach was to work cooperatively and positively with the providers to solve problems. When specific problems arose that reflected the need for special training, Triage conducted in-service programs for the providers (e.g., a program on ostomy care was arranged for the visiting nurse associations). When a conflict arose between a provider and a particular client, Triage became a mediator for problem resolution, and used its influence without taking responsibility and accountability away from the provider. Triage did not attempt to control the provider; rather it tried to help solve conflicts without sacrificing client needs. For the sake of continued good will and cooperation, it was important to have the rights of both the provider and the consumer respected.

Triage worked with each provider to develop a reporting procedure which was consonant with the provider's particular system. This effort was important in the continuing relationship between Triage and its providers because it showed the providers that someone was paying attention to their needs. Providers could be sure that they were not performing services in isolation. Triage, when appropriate, was supportive of provider decisions, a situation that often contrasted favorably with the relationship between the provider and the traditional reimbursement experience.

There were other benefits to the Triage-provider relationship. For example, supported by Triage's position of authority and responsibility, the home health agencies were able to take risks that were more consonant with their clients' needs. Sometimes when clients were able to do more for themselves than they were willing to try, Triage was able to apply its independent perspective. Thus, Triage was able to ask the visiting nurse associations or other providers to cut back on their services in order to help a client to attain more of his or her potential for independent living. With support from Triage, the providing agencies could act in the best interests of the client without fear of recrimination. If a client insisted on services that the Triage staff felt were inappropriate, the client had to assume the responsibility of paying for them.

Triage became totally familiar with its providers. It knew their capabilities and was able to capitalize on them, as it did, for example, in contracting with nursing homes for a segment of the meals-on-wheels program. The providers themselves became aware of their potential for increasing services to the community. They were able to communicate with and give support to one another. They became more than providers of isolated services—they became part of a team working for the same goals, responsible not only to their clients but to the community as a whole.

The providers that served Triage clients ranged from the highly complex modern hospital to independent "friendly visitors" and chore-workers, and were representative of the mix of volunteer, non-profit voluntary, public proprietary, and commercial sectors which characterize the American health-care marketplace. This mixture is necessary to create a system of comprehensive services that is flexible and responsive to older Americans.

Triage coordinated provider efforts in delivering eight major types of services:

- institutional,
- ambulatory,
- ancillary medical services,
- home health,
- mental health,
- social support,
- transportation, and
- meals-on-wheels.

A discussion of provider relations in the process of developing and coordinating each of these types of service follows, including a description of what providers were available, what programs had to be developed, what problems were encountered, and how these probelms were resolved.

Institutional Services

Institutional services were provided by hospitals, skilled nursing facilities (SNF's), intermediate care facilities (ICF's), and homes for the aged.

With four hospitals in the region, and contracts with eight additional facilities outside the region, hospital bed availability was assured. However, the problem of cooperation did provide a measure of difficulty. Many hospitals had initiated home care programs which focus on the immediate needs of recently discharged patients. The Triage project was designed to complement those programs and to act as a partner in the process of providing health care for the elderly. Certain hospital programs, however, perceived the project as competition, as unnecessary duplication of service, or as interference in their process. Lack of cooperation in one specific case became a deliberate attempt to impede the coordination and monitoring process through refusal to provide Triage with the paperwork necessary for implementing care planning or delivery of service. Triage was able to solve this problem by working around the home-care coordinator of the one hospital and establishing close communication with the hospital's social service department, which was willing to fill out the necessary forms and share the needed information.

Although hospital beds were always in adequate supply, a shortage in the number of nursing home beds developed. This shortage sometimes meant that Triage was not able to match a particular client with a particular facility. However, no client was ever denied care in a skilled nursing facility for lack of a bed.

Triage insisted that its clients receive the kind of care a skilled nursing facility is licensed to provide, in accordance with the "conditions of participation." Conflict could and did occur when homes were understaffed, so that care was not always of the highest quality. Cost is a major factor in perpetuating the negative conditions that exist in many nursing homes. Because Medicare will only reimburse a skilled nursing facility for certain kinds of services dealing with specific medical problems, only those services are routinely provided. Other services, especially those that address psychosocial needs, are often just as important to the patient's overall health as are traditional medical services. However, because such services are not reimbursed, they are not provided.

Much of the care that was delivered in nursing homes ran counter to the Triage goal of having each client attain the highest possible level of independent living. Institutional efficiency was a prime culprit in perpetuating client dependency. It was easier and less expensive in terms of manpower costs to perform activities (dressing and feeding, for example) for patients than to assign someone to encourage them to take care of themselves. It was much faster to feed an aged person than to stand by and watch him/her struggle with a spoon; and it was faster to dress someone than to watch him/her fumble with buttons and zippers. For the sake of efficiency, patients were cared for in a way that would best suit the operational schedule of the institution. In the name of efficiency, dignity and independence were sacrificed. Instead of the institution's meeting the needs of the patient, the patient was meeting the needs of the institution.

Another factor that created institutional dependency was the nursing home staff's attitude toward patient placement. In many cases it was simply assumed that once a patient entered a nursing home, he/she was there for the rest of his/her life. That being the case, there was no incentive to spend time encouraging independence.

Triage worked with nursing homes to improve their quality of care. Because Triage, with its unique funding arrangement, was able to obtain waivered services for its clients, nursing homes could be reimbursed for services which previously had been restricted. With money available, Triage was able to negotiate with the homes and work with them to provide the full-range, individualized kind of care that the clients needed. Moreover, as Triage had as its general goal the returning of clients to a home setting whenever possible, the nursing staff was reoriented to encourage independent functioning. Triage monitored treatment to ensure that each patient was receiving only as much nursing help as he or she required. The result was that clients would reach their maximum potential for independent functioning even if they were never able to leave the institution.

Although the majority of Triage clients who received nursing home care were in skilled nursing facilities, a few were in intermediate care facilities. An intermediate care facility is a nursing home that provides limited nursing supervision and care for patients who do not require care in a hospital or skilled nursing facility. In most cases, comprehensive home care services can substitute for the intermediate level of care. As a result, intermediate care facilities were rarely needed for Triage clients.

The third type of nursing home available to Triage clients was the home for the aged. A home for the aged is a facility that provides personal and/or protective care on a long-term basis for residents who do not require continuous nursing care but who do require assistance in performing activities of daily living. Although homes for the aged were in adequate supply, Triage clinicians generally did not prescribe them for their clients. One of the reasons for this was that a trend had developed to deinstitutionalize the mentally retarded and mentally ill by placing them in homes for the aged. These populations tended to be much younger and much more disturbed than were the Triage clients. In general, this situation created an environment not conducive to the well-being of the elderly patient, one in which the ability of the institution to deliver essential services had become severely taxed.

Day care became available through a contract signed with a licensed, non-profit, multilevel geriatric facility located about 20 miles away from the Triage service area. This was, however, another service type that was rarely used by Triage clients. There were several reasons why day care was not often selected. In most cases, either institutional care at the skilled-nursing-facility level or home-based services were deemed more appropriate. Moreover, the use of day care was limited by the transportation problem resulting from the relatively long distance between the day care center and the Triage area.

Foster homes did not exist in the region, and Triage did not encourage their development. The Triage staff believed that it would be difficult for an elderly person to move into someone else's home. While the use of foster homes could have alleviated some problems, it was conceivable that the stress it created could well have outweighed any benefit that might have been derived. The Triage administrative staff decided the demand would not be great enough to warrant the amount of time and effort which would be required to establish and monitor quality foster homes.

Ambulatory Services

For those clients whose health problems could be treated without institutionalization, ambulatory care was provided by physicians, dentists, podiatrists, audiologists and hearing aid dealers, optometrists, opticians, and physical and speech therapists. Other ambulatory service providers included pharmacies, laboratories, and medical equipment and supply companies.

Physician's services were available through hospital outpatient clinics as well as through private practices. Triage did not have a contractual arrangement with physicians. These providers performed their services under Medicare Part A, Part B, and Medicaid regulations. Over 300 different physicians served the Triage population. Although some shortages of primary care practitioners occurred at the individual level, the area itself had a sufficient supply. However, difficulties were often encountered in obtaining those services.

Several factors made adequate care in hospital clinics particularly difficult for the homebound elderly. One of the factors was the early hour at which the clinics opened. To ensure that they would be seen by the physician on a particular day, the patients had to arrive when the clinic first opened. Unfortunately, it often proved difficult for the elderly clients to be ready at such an early hour. Moreover, once patients arrived at the clinic, they often had to endure long hours of waiting.

Another problem was the rotating clinic schedule; a different physician might be on duty each day. This situation created a loss of continuity and a depersonalization of care that inhibited a doctor's ability to assess the patient's physical condition and needs. In spite of the higher cost, it was usually preferable for a client to go to a private physician, who could familiarize him or herself with the client's problems and take a personal interest in his or her care.

Triage was able to surmount the difficulties in securing care from private physicians by providing transportation for clients and by persuading more local physicians, particularly those just establishing their practices, to make house calls. However, other problems arose. Although Triage encouraged physicians to accept the Medicare assignment rate of payment for their services, some categorically refused, while others selectively determined those clients for whom they would accept this method of reimbursement. One major reason for their reluctance was that the reimbursement rates under Medicare were generally much lower than the physicians' customary fees. In addition, the traditional system requires the provider who accepts assignment to submit multiple claims, to both the patient and supplemental insurers, for coinsurance and deductible remainders which are frequently less than the collection effort costs. Thus, it may be simpler and more economical to refuse assignment, bill the patient the charge, and leave the patient to deal with Medicare and his other insurers. This gives rise to uncollected or overdue accounts and conflict between the provider and patient. Triage, with its single entry billing system, offered a streamlined reimbursement process. As the project matured, many physicians came to accept assignment for Triage clients because their lower fees were more than compensated for by the fact that they had to bill only one source—Triage—and were thereby generally assured of timely payment.

Another problem developed when doctors had difficulty in relating to a client. Sometimes the spoken or nonspoken attitude toward the elderly patient's complaints was that his or her problems were just a natural consequence of aging, and that the patient would simply have to adjust. Triage staff worked with area physicians as advocates of their elderly clientele. They succeeded in making the physicians more sensitive to the needs of the elderly and more receptive and tolerant in their treatment of them.

Still other problems arose over the professional relationship between the physicians and the nurse-clinicians. The master's degree program for a nurse-clinician qualifies him/her to assess a person's physical condition and psychosocial functioning. He/she is also prepared to perform in an administrative capacity, coordinating and monitoring the delivery of health care services. Ironically, reimbursement regulations have forced the role of health care planner and authorizing agent on the physician, whose area of expertise is in the diagnosis and prescription of treatment for specific diseases, not in the mastery of the kinds of services and the administrative technicalities that are encountered in today's complex health care system. Despite their general aversion to case management, some physicians considered the new master nurse-clinician, with his/her increased authority and responsibility, a "new breed" that threatened their authority. However, the majority of physicians in the area came to recognize that, by assisting in assessment and in administering the delivery of a coordinated health care program, the nurse-clinician can free physicians to fulfill the role for which they were trained, and can help free them from the government regulations that complicate their professional lives.

Triage found that dental services to the elderly, when delivered at all, often consisted of pulling and plating. This practice worked to the detriment of the general health of the older person. Untreated dental problems were often not only painful but posed a risk of local and systemic infection. The procedure of extracting teeth and replacing them with difficult-to-fit dentures resulted in a loss of chewing function which, in some cases, could have been avoided if the remaining good teeth had been saved and more stable prosthetics provided. This loss in many cases adversely affected the nutrition of the elderly person, with a resultant decline in his or her general health. Because the other types of treatment needed to maintain oral health were more costly, and third-party coverage of dental services was minimal, too often the criterion in performing dental services was expediency rather than optimum dental care.

Dentists provided Triage clients with a variety of services, from general diagnostic, preventive, restorative, and prosthodontic care to specialized care including oral surgery, periodontics, and endodontics. Triage monitored the procedures done for appropriateness and provided reimbursement to dentists according to the dental charge screens of private insurance companies.

Triage found that there was a problem of access to many dental offices. In one town, not one dentist had an accessible first floor office. As there was little that could be done about changing this situation Triage had to refer its handicapped clients to dentists in other towns who had ground floor offices or to those who practiced in buildings where elevators or other features made their offices more accessible.

The problem of accessibility did not arise in the case of podiatrists, who also provided essential services to the clientele. The supply of podiatrists in the seven-town region was adequate to meet client needs, and the majority of providers were willing to make home visits.

Audiologists and hearing aid dealers provided vital services to elderly clients with impaired hearing. While insuring that clients who needed hearing aids could obtain them, Triage staff also guarded against inappropriate utilization. Prior to the purchase of a hearing aid, Triage required that a client be evaluated by an ear, nose, and throat specialist or audiologist to be sure that such a device would be helpful.

In raising consumer awareness of the hard-sell tactics of door-to-door hearing aid salesmen, Triage provided a service for the hearing-impaired elderly that affected their pocketbooks, as well as their hearing. Another service which helped control costs was the development of a recycling program for hearing aids. In this program, used hearing aids were sent to a company for cleaning and repair and were then resold at a substantially lower price than new ones would have cost.

Besides coordinating service for the hearing-impaired on an individual level, Triage, in cooperation with the State Commission on the Deaf and Hearing-Impaired, developed a program to train service deliverers in problems of the hearing-impaired and ways to facilitate adjustments to hearing loss.

Eye care was provided to Triage clients by either ophthalmologists (M.D.'s) or optometrists (O.D.'s), and glasses were provided by optometrists and opticians. One problem was that the reimbursement for eyeglasses was based on the Medicaid (Title XIX) rate, a rate so low that few opticians would sign contracts with Triage. (No contracts were required for optometrists.) As a result, a co-payment mechanism was established whereby Triage paid the Medicaid rate and the client paid the balance. Nonetheless, as the price of eyeglasses varied greatly from provider to provider, Triage did advise its clients to purchase them from the source that charged the most reasonable prices.

Physical therapy services were delivered to Triage clients by three types of providers: the independent practitioner, the employee of a home-health agency or nursing home, or the therapist in a group practice. While therapists in non-profit agencies such as hospitals, nursing homes, or home-health agencies provided the majority of physical therapy services to Triage clients, it was sometimes necessary to use other therapists.

Generally, physical therapy services were satisfactory when delivered in the client's home. However, a serious problem arose when physical therapy was provided as an ancillary service in nursing homes. Patients sometimes did not receive care soon enough, and sometimes their therapy sessions were not long enough. Furthermore, Triage was sometimes billed for services which were never ordered. In other cases, double billing occurred; the nursing home would bill both Triage and the client for the same physical therapy services. To resolve these issues, Triage staff visited each nursing home in question and obtained an agreement that a plan of therapy, including goals and objectives, had to be submitted to the nurse-clinician for approval before services could be initiated. This therapy plan had clearly defined, time-limited goals. Triage monitored the services carefully for quantity and quality of treatment. Triage would not allow its clients to fall into the all too common routine in which physical therapy can continue *ad infinitum*, regardless of its benefits. At the end of the defined period of time, Triage staff evaluated the client's progress. If no improvement was seen, the therapy was discontinued. When questions arose about treatments, a physical therapist consultant reviewed the case.

In addition to physical therapists, Triage also worked with speech therapists to try to restore the language function of aphasic clients. As in the case of physical therapy, goals for speech therapy were defined and time-limited.

Ancillary Medical Services

Ancillary medical services such as prescription drugs, supplies and equipment, and laboratory tests were available in the region prior to the start of Triage in 1974. They were not, however, delivered in a manner which took the special needs of the elderly into consideration.

With direction from Triage, pharmacists were able to improve the services they provided to the elderly. For example, many pharmacies were persuaded to package their medications in ways that would be more convenient for the older person. These conveniences included caps which could be easily removed by arthritic hands, labels with letters large enough for myopic eyes to read, and special packaging of dosages to assist those with a fallible memory. Many pharmacists were interested and willing to help educate the clients to better understand the medications that they were taking. In addition Triage staff instructed pharmacists to state the amount and frequency of dosage on medicine containers and on bills sent to Triage.

To promote continuity of treatment, Triage asked each client to choose one provider for all pharmaceutical needs. To this same end pharmacists were encouraged to keep a medication profile on each client. They also were encouraged to develop their clinical skills and to communicate directly with the nurse-clinician as one professional to another, rather than communicating only through the physician.

The outpatient departments of nine hospitals performed much of the diagnostic testing for Triage clients. A majority of this testing was done by an acute care hospital that had a mobile lab unit. Because of the high volume and a geographic constraint, it was also necessary to contract with proprietary laboratories for home testing.

Medical equipment and supply companies performed an important ancillary service for the client who was not institutionalized. Twelve commerical companies had contracts to provide Triage clients with oxygen, ostomy supplies, hospital beds, wheelchairs, crutches, walkers, safety devices such as tub bars, and other supplies.

Under the influence of Triage, the equipment companies became more sensitive to the needs of the elderly. Partly in response to Triage's concern that more expertise was necessary for determining what kind of equipment was most suitable for a particular client, one company even hired a nurse-consultant.

Triage also shared its expertise with providers of disposable supplies. These providers often requested advice on adapting their products to meet the special needs of the elderly.

Home Health Services

Home health agencies, primarily visiting nurse associations and public health nursing associations, are the backbone of any health services delivery model which seeks to reduce dependency on high-technology, institution-based services. When Triage was started in 1974, the quality of care delivered by these non-profit, voluntary, home health agencies was, in general, high. Nevertheless, some problems did develop.

One of the problems was that of role definition. Although in almost every instance the visiting nurses cooperated fully with Triage, on occasion, conflict developed between the nurse-clinicians and the supervisors of the visiting nurse associations. The supervisors, in some cases, felt the nurse-clinician was duplicating their function. However, the supervisors of the visiting nurse agencies lacked knowledge about other resources, especially those dealing with social needs. The result was that, although hands-on care was of a high quality, there was often poor follow-up on referrals to non-health-care agencies, to the detriment of the client. Triage worked with the supervisors of the visiting nurse associations to help them understand the role of the nurse-clinicians. The Triage nurse-clinicians would allow these supervisors to focus their attention on their most important role, that of overseeing the visiting nurses to ensure that the highest quality of skilled nursing care was being delivered. Moreover, as greater reimbursement for a wider spectrum of services became available through Triage, the visiting nurse associations found that they were able to become more creative in providing a holistic approach to meet the varied home health care needs of their elderly clients.

Other concerns related to limitations in the scope and availability of the services provided. Home health agencies provided home health aide services, skilled nursing care, and supervision. Homemaker services, physical, occupational, and speech therapy, and medical social service also were offered by some agencies. However, not all agencies provided all these services. Some agencies were limited to homemaking. Others concentrated on skilled nursing and home health aide services. Chore and companion services were virtually nonexistent. Moreover, agencies did not provide continuous, round-the-clock coverage.

To meet the increased demand for chore and companion services, Triage encouraged the visiting nurse associations to expand their scope by providing these services. Two agencies agreed to this idea and did expand their services in 1977. In an effort to meet the need for better coverage, Triage established its own round-the-clock answering service by keeping one of its clinical teams on call during off-business hours. It also assisted the five visiting nurse associations that operated in the seven-town region in submitting a joint grant proposal to the State Department of Health for experimentation with a 24-hour, seven-day-per-week program for home health care.

In addition to utilizing the services of voluntary home health agencies, Triage was obliged to contract with proprietary agencies because they did offer continuous service. However, the demand for homemaker services was so great that it could not be met even with the cooperation of the proprietary agencies. One of the solutions to this manpower shortage was to contract with individuals who would function as independent providers.

Triage monitored homemaker care for quality and appropriateness. In some instances, poor homemaker training was a problem. Sometimes, when a proprietary agency was involved, there was minimal supervision of care. Moreover, at times a profit-oriented agency would provide more care than was necessary. Triage worked with the agencies to find solutions to these problems and to assist them in delivering the care that was best for each client.

Triage signed contracts with five agencies and several individuals to perform chore services. Chore services provided to Triage clients included outdoor work such a snow shoveling and lawn mowing, as well as heavy household tasks that homemakers would not do, such as washing windows and floors and making minor repairs.

The main problem Triage encountered in providing choreworkers was that the supply of manpower was inadequate. Cost was also a concern. Established maintenance agencies did good work, for the most part, but charged prohibitive prices for their services. Sometimes even independent choreworkers charged fees that were unreasonable for the services that were rendered. Moreover, services were not always reliably performed. Sometimes the teenagers who were hired as chore-workers lacked the necessary commitment to follow through with their assigned tasks, causing hardships to the clients. If a client's sidewalk did not get shoveled, for example, that client would have great difficulty getting to and from his house. Triage worked to develop a pool of reliable providers who would charge reasonable fees for their services.

Triage employed the services of several independent companions. Sometimes these companions were used because the agencies did not have enough available staff to meet client needs; companions would often work in the evening when homemakers and home health aides were not available. At other times, in contracting with a particular companion, Triage was formalizing a relationship which had already been initiated by the client. Triage often enlisted interested relatives, friends, or other individuals as companions to assist the client to remain in, or to return to, the community. Providers, wherever possible, were non-professionals who were residents of neighborhoods in which the clients resided.

Companions performed duties similar to those of the homemaker or the home health aide: housekeeping, cooking, unskilled nursing care, and other services the elderly person might require. The number of hours worked varied from a few hours a month for escort services to 24-hours a day, seven days a week for live-in companionship.

To meet the home health care needs of its elderly clientele, Triage found itself in a position of having to find, and often to train, people who could deliver the services it prescribed. The happy result was that Triage brought a secondary benefit to the seven-town region. Not only did it work to prescribe, coordinate, and monitor services for the elderly, but it also created many jobs which gave employment opportunities to the unemployed and the developmentally disabled, as well as to some minimally disturbed young people.

As a project dedicated to meeting the health care needs of the elderly, Triage was also sensitive to the needs of other groups struggling to attain and maintain human potential. Triage created job opportunities for the developmentally disabled by helping a sheltered vocational training organization to establish a training program for homemakers. After being trained in meal preparation, chore service, and lawn mowing, several of these individuals were hired by home health agencies in the area.

Mental Health Services

While at least a modicum of the physical needs of the elderly were being met by medical and home health services when Triage enrolled its first client, there was a dearth of home-delivered mental health services. The Triage project stimulated the community mental health center in the region to hire a staff member who specialized in mental health problems of the aging. However, this resource alone could not adequately provide the counseling in coping which so many Triage clients needed. Therefore, Triage developed contracts with independent mental health counselors for this service. The independent counselors were trained in social work, nursing, educational counseling, and clinical psychology. The emphasis on counseling rather than on psychiatric treatment was especially important to this generation of older adults who, by and large, were unreceptive to traditional psychiatric methods.

Problems with mental health counselors arose over their reluctance to make home visits, their perfunctory method of handling monthly reports, and their unwillingness to provide discharge summaries and to cooperate in the overall coordination of the care plan. Triage insisted that any mental health treatment provided for its clients have clearly-defined goals and be time-limited. Unproductive therapy was not allowed to continue forever.

Social Support Services

While some social support services were available in the region in 1974, the local agencies focused primarily on the problems of the adolescent and the younger adult population. It became necessary for Triage to help develop social support services specifically geared to the special needs of the elderly, or if these efforts were unsuccessful, to deliver support services directly.

One important service performed by Triage was that of finding housing for its clients. Housing needs for the elderly were acute and special housing for the elderly was at a premium when Triage started in 1974. Often people were placed on waiting lists for five to six years. The three basic types of housing available to the elderly were low-income public housing, elderly housing under the auspices of the local housing authority, and non-profit sponsored elderly housing. In general, elderly housing was much more desirable than low-income housing because it was designed to meet the specific needs of the elderly and to be easier to maintain. It also provided a better, safer environment. Unfortunately, administrative procedures often thwarted a person who sought elderly housing. The non-profit agencies provided housing for elderly persons who had higher incomes. Although their procedures were much more flexible than those of the local housing authorities, the agencies also had many eligibility restrictions. Persons with serious health care problems were discouraged, as were people in wheelchairs. Triage had to become an advocate for its clients, pleading the case of each individual on the basis of need and that person's capacity to function independently.

Triage staff also informed their clients, many of whom would not otherwise have been aware, of tax relief procedures such as the elderly freeze that made it more feasible for some people to remain in their own homes. The elderly freeze refers to the practice, followed by many towns in Connecticut, of freezing property taxes at the rate in effect the year the owner turns 65 years of age, thus protecting the elderly from future rate increases. Triage assisted them in negotiating the procedures necessary for obtaining the rebates, a financial settlement that sometimes proved to be rather substantial.

Besides locating housing, Triage helpled the elderly maintain their homes by developing a private fund, with contributions from local churches, which paid for emergency repairs. In a related area, Triage staff began negotiations with the Department of Housing and Urban Development (HUD) to provide halfway housing to nursing home residents who desired to return to the community. They also worked with the State Departments on Aging and Community Affairs in developing guidelines for congregate housing.

Triage took advantage of the fact that many of its clients attended senior centers regularly to enlist the cooperation of the centers in providing some health services for those who used the facilities. When a new center opened in the fall of 1975, Triage developed an instrument to assess the health of the elderly clientele, and helped the visiting nurses set up a weekly health clinic at the senior center.

Besides its involvement with the clinic, Triage cooperated with senior centers in many different ways. Many Triage clients participated in the congregate meal programs provided at the centers. Often, the centers would refer clients who were considered in need of Triage services. In addition, Triage was instrumental in starting a Tai-Chi program through which the elderly could enjoy the benefits of the ancient form of Chinese exercise.

Triage, as an advocate of the elderly, performed an important social support service. Triage social service coordinators became extensively involved in ensuring that their clients received the services for which they were eligible under Titles XVIII and XIX of the Social Security Act and Titles III and VII of the Older Americans Act. They also often interceded to ensure that the clients, if entitled, received such benefits as food stamps, elderly housing, and tax rebates.

Social isolation, besides being a problem to the client himself, presented a problem for Triage in determining and meeting the needs of some of its elderly clients, particularly those residing in rural areas. To solve this problem, Triage helped mobilize the voluntary sector to recruit and train friendly visitors and to implement telephone reassurance programs. Triage team members worked to train elderly volunteers to perform this important communication function. These volunteers were trained in the needs and behavior patterns of socially isolated people. Their role was to provide regular human contact for the isolated person. By telephone or in person, the volunteers would simply talk to the elderly person to stimulate him mentally and keep him in touch with the world around him. This valuable service let the person know that he was not all alone, that there was someone who cared, and that there was still some order and meaning to life. An effort was made to match the interests and personalities of the visitors to those of the clients. Though not paid, the friendly visitors were reimbursed for their transportation expenses.

Transportation

Special transportation services for the elderly were almost non-existent prior to 1976. Because transportation was a crucial link in obtaining necessary medical and social services, Triage made special arrangements with various providers to meet the needs of its clients, whether the need was for an ambulance, a chair car, a taxi, or a van.

Seven ambulance and chair car companies had contracts with Triage. Ambulances provided vital emergency transportation to hospitals and also provided a means of moving bedridden clients. However, outside of emergency situations, ambulances were unreliable, often causing clients much needless anxiety and inconvenience by making them wait long beyond the appointed time.

Chaircars were used to meet the special transportation needs of those clients who were confined to wheelchairs (or who needed wheelchairs if they had to travel an appreciable distance).

Triage negotiated contracts with each of the taxi companies in the seven-town region, thereby providing mobility for many of the elderly who, because of their limited incomes, could not previously afford to take taxis. The taxi companies that provided transportaton for Triage clients were all proprietary and were regulated in rates and standards by the Public Utilities Commission Authority (PUCA).

The long waiting time was not the only problem. Some taxi companies had regulations that prevented them from crossing town lines. Some cab drivers expressed annoyance at the reduced mobility of many Triage clients. Moreover, on more than one occasion, taxi drivers took advantage of their elderly passengers. Triage staff tried to resolve these difficulties with the providers. By making them more aware of the needs of the elderly, Triage hoped that the providers would become more sensitive to and tolerant of the clients. Sometimes, to facilitate travel by taxi, an escort was provided.

The rural areas especially lacked transportation resources. However, Triage was able to hire a van operated by a volunteer program to travel one day each week to the rural housing complex to transport people to shopping centers, banks, or physicians' offices. In addition, volunteer agencies assisted in providing transportation for the elderly under the stipulations of their own organizations. Triage also provided the shut-in elderly with weekly transportation for socialization. To minimize costs, Triage made transportation arrangements with agencies that operated vans. Unfortunately, the demand for their services was greater than their capacity to provide it. As a result, Triage had to rely on commercial providers such as taxi companies that charged the going rate.

Meals-On-Wheels

Meals-on-wheels programs, like transportation services for the elderly, were lacking in the seven-town region prior to 1974. At that time, the only facility which operated a small meals-on-wheels program was a local hospital.

Because no one agency would assume responsiblitiy for the entire operation, it was necessary to contract with two separate agencies—one for each of the two stages of the operation: preparation and delivery. However, these agencies were unable to service all seven towns. To extend meal service to the entire region, Triage enlisted the cooperation of additional providers, including convalescent homes, catering services, and restaurants.

In addition to meeting the needs of its own clients, Triage also encouraged the providers to serve meals to needy elderly persons who were not Triage clients. Toward this end, Triage negotiated with the Department of Agriculture to enable non-clients to pay for home-delivered meals with food stamps. Constraints in the food stamp legislation prevented this arrangement from being implemented. The problem of providing high quality home-delivered meals in sufficient quantity remained a Triage concern. As no standards or regulations existed for meals-on-wheels programs, Triage hired a nutritional consultant who helped to establish standards of quality and quantity and to set up rotating diet schedules. The majority of the providers complied with the project's standards. Triage monitored meal services by performing spot checks for quality control.

Some difficulties were experienced in the delivery of the meals. Because the job of meal delivery was low paying, provider commitment and reliability were sometimes lacking. Triage staff found it necessary to meet with the deliverers of the meals on a regular basis to educate them as to the vital importance of their roles.

In addition to securing basic meals-on-wheels services, Triage also worked with its providers in developing the ability to prepare and distribute special diet meals for those who, because of diabetes, circulatory problems, or other conditions or preferences, had to observe dietary restrictions.

An Integrated Service Delivery System

A comprehensive approach to health care based on individual need requires that a wide range of providers be found to develop a complete spectrum of services, and that good working relationships be established with these providers. Further, these working relationships must be constantly nourished as the individuals delivering client services and the agency boards of directors change. Coordination is always more easily said than done, but Triage has demonstrated that the eight disparate types of medical and social services can be welded into an organic whole that is greater than the sum of its parts.

Claims Processing: Triage as Fiscal Intermediary

The innovative nature of the way Triage implemented the waivers and related to providers required that Triage, in cooperation with the Division of Direct Reimbursement, serve as its own fiscal intermediary and process claims in a new way.

As was indicated in the discussion of contracts, a single intermediary, the Division of Direct Reimbursement (DDR) of the Social Security Administration, was selected for the project. Its functions were to issue payments for claims processed and approved by Triage, to collect and code cost data, and to provide technical assistance in the administration of cost-related reimbursement.

The use of a single intermediary provided several advantages to the project. Triage was defining new coverage and reimbursement ground rules. A Triage claim, therefore, could not be processed through the same review procedures that were used to process ordinary Medicare bills. It would not meet definitions of coverage that would assure its successful transport through the Medicare claims network. Furthermore, the Social Security Administration would have found it difficult and costly to revise the Medicare system to accommodate the relatively small number of bills generated by the 3,000 potential Triage clients.

The claims processing function was designed to be a supportive extension of the clinical staff's frontline determination of appropriate services. The teams and the claims processing staff had the same understanding of the boundaries of the waivers and the terms of the contracts that had been negotiated with the providers. By being housed in the same location, the claims review staff and the clinical staff that authorized services had the advantage of being able to resolve problems more easily, thus helping to serve clients more effectively and to maintain good provider relations.

The service authorization, claims review, and payment process took place at Triage as follows: A nurse-clinician/social service coordinator team, upon completing an assessment, drafted a care plan and contacted providers directly to order services. As a followup to the verbal contact, a written authorization was then sent to the provider to confirm the service, limits of service, and rates. Copies of the authorization were retained at Triage, one being kept by the appropriate clinical team and the other by the claims review staff. When a provider sent a bill to Triage, the claims staff checked the bill against the authorization. If the two documents did not agree, the team was notified. The team then contacted the client and/or the provider to resolve the difference. If the claim could be processed, it was forwarded to Triage's fiscal intermediary which issued a check for the authorized service.

The claims and reimbursement process was an important staff function at Triage that took an increasingly greater amount of time. Growth in the number of clients caused a corresponding increase in the number of claims. During 1976, the number of claims received and processed was 24,000, from a caseload of 824 clients. In 1977, 46,934 claims were paid and in 1978, the total was 55,558. Over this period, the average yearly volume of claims per client remained relatively stable at about 16.9 claims per client per year.

Conclusion

Triage put into practice four of the coordination mechanisms proposed at the Regional Public Hearings on Home Health Care (September 20–October 1, 1976): a single locus of service, a coordination management mechanism, formal interagency contracts, and expansion of service agencies.

Through these mechanisms, the providers became aware of their potential for increasing services to the community. They were able to communicate with and give support to one another. They became more than providers of isolated services—they became part of a team working for the same goals, responsible not only to their clients (or their reimbursers) but to the community as a whole.

The efficient, carefully controlled claims and reimbursement system that Triage developed contributed greatly to the success of the project in both its research and service aspects. With its single funding source and its single entry billing system, Triage was a dramatic departure from the fragmented system of health care reimbursement that is the rule in traditional health care programs. Its uniform claims department procedures made it simpler for providers to bill for services and easier for clients to understand their bills. Under the Triage system, providers were also made more accountable for the services they delivered than was previously the case. However, because they were treated fairly by the claims and reimbursement system and were paid in a timely fashion, Triage's relationship with its providers was a good one that was reflected in the high quality of services that were delivered to the elderly people that Triage served.

4

Assessment of the Older Adult: A Holistic Approach

CHRISTINE JOHNSON, R.N., M.S.
NANCY RYAN, R.N., M.S.
JOAN QUINN, R.N., M.S.

Assessment is the foundation of any coordinated system of care that attempts to tailor services to individual client needs. Just as the Triage reimbursement mechanism, as described in Chapter 3, provides a single-entry system for the financing of services, the Triage assessment provides a single-entry system for the organization of comprehensive health and social services.

The assessment instrument developed by Triage is the primary vehicle through which a care plan built around individual client need is activated. The instrument incorporates the project's holistic approach to assessment—an approach that recognizes the reciprocal influences of physical, psychological, social, and economic factors on the health of the individual. This approach is in accord with Lawton's (1971) definition that assessment is the " . . . systematic attempt to measure objectively the level at which a person is functioning, in any of a variety of areas such as physical health, quality of self-maintenance, quality of role activity, intellectual status, social attitude toward the world and self, and emotional status."

The Triage assessment instrument provides a guide for both an extensive health interview and a modified physical examination. The interview includes a complete health history, measures of functioning status, and social, psychological, and economic items. The physical examination provides a complete review of organ systems.

No assessment instrument, regardless of how comprehensive and how well-constructed, is effective unless those who administer it are capable of using it correctly. The necessity for professional personnel to administer the assessment cannot be stressed enough. Because the decisions made on the basis of information derived through the assessment have far-reaching consequences, to delegate such a comprehensive evaluation to other than highly professional personnel is to do a disservice to the older person being assessed (Quinn & Ryan, 1979).

The Triage assessment is administered by a nurse-clinician and social worker team, who have the necessary professional training to evaluate the complex range of problems which the older person may present. The nurse-clinician's knowledge and experience integrate nursing theory with medicine, mental health, social services, nutrition, and rehabilitative therapy. The social worker's knowledge and experience include case management, counseling, and community organization.

Because the assessment instrument is the basis for the care plan, it is preferable that the same professionals who will coordinate and monitor the plan conduct the initial assessment. Whenever possible, the assessment is scheduled so that both members of the team can participate in the initial interview. The participation of both nurse and social worker not only results in a more comprehensive evaluation of the client, but also establishes the team concept with the client at the start. On those occasions when the team is unable to make a joint visit, the assessment is done by the nurse alone because she is capable of administering the entire instrument, including the extensive medical history and physical examination. However, in no case is a care plan developed without consultation with the social worker.

The setting in which the assessment takes place is the client's home. Only in the home setting is it possible for the assessor to observe the client's interaction with his or her environment. On occasion, an assessment may be done in a nursing home or hospital if there is evidence that the client's institutionalization is only temporary. In those cases, a home visit is made after the client has been discharged to evaluate the home environment.

While the time required to complete the assessment will depend on the attention span and degree of fragility of the older person, it generally takes about one and one-half hours. When this amount of time is a burden on the client, the completion of the interview is postponed for a return visit. If the client has a mentation or communication problem, another informant, such as a family member or a health professional already involved in the case, may be called upon to answer some of the questions.

Some might argue that the assessment instrument is too lengthy, but Triage has found that the expenditure of time during the initial assessment saves time in ensuing encounters with the older person. It must be remembered that simple yes/no questions are not being asked. The questions are intended to elicit meaningful information which, often having been stored for over 65 years, requires time to explore.

Before the assessment instrument is administered, the team tries to establish an initial rapport with the elderly person. The individual is thoroughly informed about the nature of the agency in general and the nature of the specific items which will be included in the interview. Only after truly informed consent is given does the assessment begin. Usually a unique, positive relationship is established at the beginning of the assessment that is invaluable in ongoing interaction with the elderly person.

To sustain this rapport, the assessment instrument is designed to flow from impersonal to more personal information. This format allows the person to become comfortable with the interviewer(s) and the assessment process before discussing potentially sensitive subjects, such as mental health or finances. These kinds of topics are generally addressed midway or toward the end of the interview.

Contents

The Triage assessment instrument contains 212 items. These items are broadly grouped into five categories—social, physical health and medical, psychological, functioning status, and economic—and then further subdivided into 28 types (see Table 4–1).

Social Items

Age, marital status, primary language, cultural background, neighborhood, and housing arrangements are some of the social items that influence the individual and must be considered when developing a

TABLE 4-1. Assessment Form Contents

Category	Items Included
I. Social Items	1. Identifying Information 2. Sociodemographic Characteristics 3. Environmental Assessment 4. Social Functioning 5. Family Support
II. Physical Health and Medical Items	6. Subjective Health Status 7. Objective 8. Medical Treatments 9. Medications 10. Allergies 11. Vision 12. Oral Health 13. Podiatric Health 14. Nutritional Assessment 15. Prior Utilization of Health Services 16. Health History 17. Family Health History 18. Symptomatology 19. Physical Exam Findings 20. Medical Problems Encountered
III. Psychological Items	21. Subjective and Objective Mental Health 22. Life Satisfaction 23. Stress Situations
IV. Functioning Status	24. Activities of Daily Living (ADL) 25. Instrumental Activities of Daily Living (IADL) 26. Mental Status Questionnaire (MSQ)
V. Economic Items	27. Income 28. Living Expenditures

care plan. Age is associated with both financial limitations and health service utilization. In an inflationary period such as ours, the purchasing power of fixed incomes declines while health expenditures rise. For example, although the elderly are only 10 percent of the population, they account for 22 percent of the utilization of hospital services. And while their medical expenses are much higher than those of other age groups, their incomes generally are considerably lower than the incomes of younger adults (Brotman, 1978). Age is also important as a cohort variable. For example, the 85-year-old male of 1980 probably served in World War I, while the 65-year-old was only an infant at the time.

The medical and epidemiological significance of gender in health care programs is well-established. Men have a shorter life span than women. Women reside in nursing homes at nearly twice the rate of men (Brody, 1970).

The relevance of marital status is demonstrably linked with many measures of morbidity and mortality (Glick, 1975). Mortality risk is higher among divorced persons than among the widowed.

Higher levels of education have been associated with relatively more medical care, especially preventive care. In addition, those who are better educated provide more care for themselves and their families or simply are more willing to follow medical advice. They also are more aware of how to seek out and select appropriate health care services (Fuchs, 1972).

Cultural backgrounds usually influence important areas of behavior such as eating habits. For example, if a nutritional problem exists due to an individual's inability to prepare meals, the meals-on-wheels program may appear to be a simple, reasonable solution. Yet a closer analysis may reveal that because of ethnic food preferences, the meals provided will not be acceptable to the client, and thus alternatives will have to be explored. Cultural background may also influence other aspects of client behavior, such as willingness to accept mental health counseling.

Another important sociodemographic characteristic is occupation/retirement. To make the appropriate assessment, the interviewer should ask: How recent was the retirement? From what occupation has the client retired? What is the effect on income? What is the effect on social relationships? Have any physical limitations occurred as the result of employment? Most of today's elderly population have been forced to retire at the age of 65, and few, if any, have had the opportunity to participate in preretirement planning programs. For some of these individuals, especially the males, retirement poses a real problem in adapting to a new lifestyle and presents a challenge to the health care provider who is developing a plan of care. The situational stresses retirees face are varied and can include a considerable drop in income, a loss of social contacts, increased time to spend with a spouse or others with whom he or she lives, lack of interests or hobbies to replace time usually occupied with work, and a predisposition to or the acquiring of a medical problem. The interviewer must determine if it is enough to introduce the client to the available resources in the community, such as the local senior center, or if there is a more deep-seated problem that requires professional treatment.

When inquiring about past occupations, the interviewer must also be alert to possible physical problems that the client may have developed over time. Often, work-related problems are not identified at their inception, have a gradual progression, and thus may be over-looked due to adaptation or simply attributed to the aging process. For instance, while progressive hearing loss may have resulted from a high noise level in the workplace, the problem may not be identified until later in life and then attributed to aging rather than to the occupational health hazard.

Environmental Assessment. The environmental assessment takes into consideration the physical surroundings in which the client resides and pertains to cleanliness as well as to the presence or absence of architectural barriers. If the client is physically impaired, the home must be evaluated in terms of the client's access to the outdoors and maneuverability within the structure. There must also be a deter-mination of the client's ability to maintain his or her environment in a safe and sanitary condition. Furthermore, the environment must be evaluated not only for the safety of the client, but also for the safety of those who come in contact with the client. (A home health aide may be unwilling to care for a client if she has to climb a dangerous staircase or work in a poorly heated home.)

The environment is one area in which it is easy for the interviewer's values to interfere with the assessment. It must be remembered that evaluation should be made in the context of the client's value system. What appears squalid to a health professional may be casual or lived-in to the client.

Living Arrangements. It is essential to determine the usual living arrangements of the client since household members must be included in any plan of care. If household members are already assisting the client, there should be no disruption in their plan of care, unless they consider this arrangement unsuccessful or incompatible with their own needs or those of the client.

The elderly person with severe physical limitations or mentation problems runs a greater risk of institutionalization if he or she lives alone. It has been found that in many instances couples are able to maintain themselves in the community for a longer period of time because the deficits of one spouse may be compensated for by the strengths of the other. Thus, the physically impaired individual can be helped physically by the confused or forgetful individual and the confused can be helped by the mentally alert individual who may be physically impaired.

Social Functioning. Among the elderly, maintenance of contacts in the social environment is essential for a sense of social well-being and life satisfaction. When social contacts are not maintained, social isolation is the result. Social isolation has been implicated as a factor in the incidence of mental illness (Lowenthal, 1965; Neugarten, Havighurst, and Tobin, 1961).

To determine the type and amount of social functioning in which the client is engaged, the assessors ask five questions concerning the frequency with which the client interacts with relatives, friends, neighbors, co-workers, and other associates. The five questions are:

1. How often do you attend group, club, or religious functions?
2. How often do you see your children?
3. How often do you see your other relatives, neighbors, and friends?
4. How often do you see people such as the visiting nurse, voluntary workers, clergy, etc.?
5. Do you work?

Family Support. The interviewers must also determine the presence or absence and strengths and weaknesses of the older person's support system, whether it be spouse, children, other relatives, friends, or neighbors. Family support incorporates many elements which are measured by seven items on the assessment instrument: living arrangements, illness of household members in the past year, health of supporter, stress on supporter, number of children in the area, frequency of social contacts, and family harmony.

In the majority of cases, the support system of an individual gives more care in the home setting than any private agency. If one were to calculate the expenditures of a family in giving care to the older person with moderate impairment, the cost might be equal to or exceed that of a long-term care facility. A recent study by the General Accounting Office (1977) reported that for clients at the most impaired levels, home-service values increase rapidly. At the extremely impaired level, families and friends were providing about $673 per month in services for every $172 being spent by agencies.

Although the personal support systems of the elderly often provide a considerable amount of care, all care givers do reach a saturation point and then need time to remove themselves temporarily from their responsibility, concentrate on themselves, and restore their energies to carry on. Often the supporter is under as much, if not more, physical and/or emotional stress as the client and needs relief for an hour, a day, or a week or two. The assessment must provide information to determine whether there is mutual desire by supporter(s) and client for the client to remain at home, and if so, what help the supporter needs in carrying out the caretaker role. The provision of adequate respite care may enable a heavily taxed support system to continue, thus decreasing the possibility of undesired institutionalization.

Physical Health and Medical Items

History and Problem List. In the medical history section of the assessment, the interviewer asks about past hospitalizations and past and current medical problems. It is the rare elderly person who has not had some sort of past medical condition. The older adult has had at least 65 years to develop a history, and it is essential to document all medical problems, whether or not they are in an acute stage.

In addition to the medical history, a review of biological systems which elicits answers to questions about symptoms is necessary. Generalized symptoms, such as feeling tired, unwell, or weak, should be documented on the assessment in the same manner as other, more specific complaints. All too often, clients will overlook non-specific symptoms, considering them to be the result of normal aging.

Triage has found that the medical problems encountered through the assessment interview are best documented according to the format of the problem-oriented record (Weed, 1971) which is ideally suited to a client-centered system. With Weed's method, every step in the management of the client's care is taken only as it relates to a specific problem in the context of all the problems on a master problem list.

A problem, as defined by Weed, has four components known by their initials as "SOAP." The first component, "S," is the subject's (client's) perception of the problem. The second component, "O," is the objective evaluation of the problem made by the trained assessor. "A," the third component, is the assessment of the problem based on the subjective and objective components. The fourth component, "P," is the plan formulated in the context of the other three components. The importance of going beyond the subjective component to the objective is illustrated in the following examples.

An elderly person who has chronic congestive heart failure with multiple hospitalizations for that problem may not view the latest acute episode as a major problem unless he or she perceives it as life threatening. Even if the client does not consider the episode as being major, the interviewer must investigate further to determine if a plan of care can be developed to decrease the number of acute episodes. It is possible that noncompliance with medications or diet, for whatever reason, may be the triggering mechanism.

Similarly, if a person does not think that a condition is interfering with his or her functional ability, in that person's mind the condition does not exist. The professional may be able to observe shortness of breath, but due to its chronicity, the client may no longer perceive it as problematic. The fact that her feet hurt at the moment and she cannot ambulate may be at the top of a client's list of problems, rather than the fact that she has difficulty breathing.

Medical Treatment. Just as a client may not perceive a medical condition as a problem unless it is life-threatening, so the client may not perceive a medical treatment as a treatment unless it is for an acute condition. It is not unusual for a person to have a ten-year history of hypertension, be on medication, and completely neglect mentioning this, because "I don't think about it . . . . I've had it so long, it doesn't bother me any longer."

Through this section of the assessment, it is also revealed that many times those individuals who are receiving treatment are not following the prescribed treatment. The reasons for noncompliance are varied. Some elderly people have so many problems that they are not clear about their various treatment plans, especially if no one has bothered to give them written instructions. Another contributing factor is that with so many problems, one treatment plan may conflict with another. (For example, a person with cardiac problems cannot always tolerate exercises that would benefit his arthritic condition.)

Medications. The main focus of this portion of the assessment is to determine all the prescribed and over-the-counter medications of the client. A major problem often encountered is the number of different drugs the elderly person takes. Drug problems arise either because the client has multiple problems that require medication or because the client is seeing several physicians for individual medical problems and none of the physicians is aware of what the others have prescribed. Triage staff have found clients who were taking as many as 17 medications when only a few were medically necessary.

Triage clients are not unique in taking multiple medications. At the turn of the century, Sir William Osler (1906) observed that human beings are distinguished from the lower orders by the proclivity to take medications. Eighty years later, Cousins (1979) repeated this observation and added that the human species might also be characterized by its ability to survive medication.

Not all medications are prescribed. Specific questioning as to use of non-prescribed, over-the-counter drugs is also necessary. Drug interactions can occur just as frequently and as seriously with over-the-counter medicines as with those drugs that are prescribed by physicians.

A secondary focus of the questions relating to medications is the schedule of administration. It is not unusual to find that a client is taking many different medications at varying times during the day. In some instances, the scheduling of dosages becomes very complex, and either the client forgets to take the medications or decides some are not important and discontinues their usage. Through the assessment, the interviewers learn whether a new schedule of administration must be developed which conforms to the client's life style. It is usually easier to achieve compliance if medications are not taken more frequently than one time per day, although sometimes divided dosages are necessary.

A third problem area addressed in this section of the assessment is that of appropriate dosage. Drug dosage must be adapted to the

individual's biological, not chronological, age and prescribed in relation
to the organ systems that metabolize the drugs. Unintended over-
dosage may result if the normal physiological and cellular changes that
occur with aging are ignored. For example, if systems for excretion are
impaired, drugs can accumulate in the body, eventually causing over-
dosage and subsequent kidney damage.

Physical Examination

In a comprehensive assessment, a modified physical examination is
important because it provides the interviewer with current baseline
data about the client acquired at first hand. For many clients this may
be the first time in many years that a thorough physical examination has
been performed. Through assessment, one finds clients who have been
taking medications, especially for hypertension and diabetes, but who
have not seen a physician for follow-up for several years.

Therefore, physical assessment should include, but not necessarily
be limited to, an examination of eyes, ears, mouth, neck, abdomen, and
cardio-pulmonary, musculoskeletal, neurological, and genitourinary
systems. It is essential for the examiner to be able to distinguish
between what is normal physiological aging and what is a pathological
condition. Positive findings should be followed up with the client and
the client's primary physician.

Dental Information

Dental care is important to nutritional intake as well as to self-concept.
It is, therefore, essential to ask if the client has difficulty chewing; if the
client has bleeding or painful gums; if the client needs dentures; or, if
the client already has dentures, whether they fit properly. The client's
apparent need for a prothesis must be carefully evaluated. Frequently,
people who have been edentulous for several years, or who have had the
same pair of dentures for 20 to 30 years, do not adjust well to new
dentures. In these situations, new dentures often end up in water-filled
glasses or a chest of drawers, not in people's mouths. If old dentures
become loose due to the changing anatomical structure of the mouth,
relining will usually adequately solve the client's problem. If the client
is not edentulous, the goal is generally to maintain the teeth for as long

as possible through regularly scheduled preventive and restorative treatment.

Nutrition

Reasons for inadequate nutrition among the elderly are numerous. Four of the most common are:

1. physical difficulty in obtaining food because of inability to carry groceries;
2. lack of desire or inability to prepare meals;
3. inadequate finances to purchase nutritious foods;
4. absence of teeth.

One must therefore ask questions from both social and physical perspectives. Who shops for food? What are the facilities for storage? Who prepares meals? How is the client's appetite? With whom does the client eat? Is there enough money for food? What is the typical day's menu? These social questions are all part of a comprehensive data base. In addition, a review of organ systems and a physical assessment are performed to determine the client's dental and gastrointestinal status and to uncover possible physical barriers to adequate nutrition.

Because a plan of care that addresses nutritional problems will vary greatly according to individual needs, the assessment of nutritional status must be comprehensive. The items mentioned above are not the only ones that could be explored, but they will assure that enough information is gathered to develop an appropriate plan. Interventions to correct nutritional deficiencies brought about because of financial or social reasons will differ greatly from interventions to address problems with a medical basis (e.g., those caused by a lack of inadequate dentition or a gastric ulcer).

Sensory Impairment

Assessment of sensory impairment is important for an accurate evaluation of the elderly. People who are unable to see and hear have perceptual difficulty and often are incorrectly labeled "confused" or "senile." With a visual deficit, an elderly person sitting at a dinner table may ask to have the mashed potatoes passed, when the vegetable is actually cauliflower. Or, the person may respond inappropriately to a question or to the conversation at hand, not because of confusion, but because he or she did not hear what was said. People with hearing and visual difficulties often intentionally withdraw from society because they are embarrassed by their deficiency. As a result, they may deprive themselves of valuable social interaction which acts as a stimulus for improved orientation to time, place, and person. Often a plan of care need simply incorporate such features as proper lighting to compensate for visual deficits. Similarly, a proper hearing aid or corrective lenses may "cure" what has been prematurely labeled "senility."

In addition to sight and hearing, the other senses, including taste, smell, and touch, should be assessed. These senses often diminish with normal physiological aging and/or pathology.

Psychological Items

Documentation of both objective and subjective mental health status is essential. Two dimensions of objective mental health are assessed: cognitive functioning and indicators of mental illness.

It is extremely important to document the individual's orientation to time and place. One valuable tool with which to measure this aspect of functioning status is the Mental Status Questionnaire (MSQ), developed by Kahn et al. (1960). This scale is short and therefore can be readministered frequently without overburdening the client.

The ten questions which comprise this scale are:

1. What is your street address?
2. Where is this place located?
3. What is today's date?
4. What is the month now?
5. What year is it?
6. How old are you?
7. What month were you born?
8. What year were you born?

9. Who is the President of the U.S.?
10. Who was the President before him?

The number of errors on this scale differentiate between degrees of severity of chronic brain syndrome: none or minimal, moderate or severe.

Although the Mental Status Questionnaire is a useful tool, it explores only one dimension of mental health, that is, cognitive functioning. In addition, the interviewer must document other indicators of mental illness, including the presence or absence of perseveration, confusion, confabulation, garrulousness, inattentiveness, loss of emotional control, aggressiveness, hostility, untidy dress, poor grooming, and food stains. It is also necessary to separate those life-long patterns of aggressiveness, hostility, untidy dress, and poor grooming that stem from personality traits or life-style from recent changes that represent mental deterioration. If the interviewer perceives that one of these symptoms is present, it is mandatory to further investigate the client's physical as well as mental status. All too often, the label of senility is attached to the elderly, with little or no evaluation of the cause of the behavior. There are many reasons for behavioral changes, and the elderly should be evaluated completely before a diagnosis is made.

In the area of subjective mental health, questions concerning morale, activity level, and mood are covered. Because the rate of suicide among the depressed elderly is high, it is of the utmost importance to note whether the elderly person is lonely, has difficulty sleeping, or experiences feelings that life is not worth living.

Life Satisfaction. The degree of life satisfaction is an important indicator of subjective mental health. Six questions are used to measure life satisfaction:

- Are you happy?
- Do you ever feel life is not worth living?
- Are you lonely?
- Do you get depressed?
- Do you worry?
- Are you comfortable where you are?

Stress. Stressful life events have been associated with susceptibility to illness, physical as well as mental (Holmes & Masuda, 1970).
Therefore, stress is another dimension of mental health measured by
the Triage instrument.

Stress was operationally defined by adapting the Geriatric Social
Readjustment Rating Scale (GSRRS) developed by Amster and Krauss
(1974). The 35 items on this scale were evaluated by the Triage clinical
and research staff and 16 were selected as being suitable for inclusion
in the Triage assessment form. The 16 items selected, adapted, and
incorporated within the Triage stress characteristic are related to seven
areas:

- death of significant others and changes in health of self or
  significant others,
- work,
- finances,
- living arrangements,
- family,
- marital status,
- sexual behavior.

The responses recorded are self-reports without objective verification.
It is important for the clinical team to assess how well the client is
coping with stress before they prescribe an intervention.

Functioning Status: ADL/IADL

Two important measures of functioning status are the Activities of
Daily Living, or ADL (Katz & Akpom, 1976), and the Instrumental
Activities of Daily Living, or IADL (Lawton & Brody, 1969). These
indices are the primary basis for determining the human assistance
needs of a client. Measured by the Activities of Daily Living index are
such functions as ability to eat, transfer, toilet, control one's bowel and
bladder, bathe, and dress. The Instrumental Activities of Daily Living
index measures the ability to use the telephone, shop, prepare food,
keep house, do the laundry, travel, take medication, and handle
finances. Assessment of these functions can determine if the individual

is independent, intermediate (dependent on some help from other persons), or totally dependent.

Economic Items

Finances. While physical, emotional, and social parameters are important in the development of a care plan, the immediate and long-range financial implications of such a plan to the client must not be ignored. Therefore, a comprehensive assessment must include a section on financial resources, obligations, and expenditures.

Basic information should be gathered on income, pension or retirement benefits, Supplemental Security Income (SSI), rental income, interest on savings, and income from other sources. However, unless' it is necessary to determine financial eligibility for services, the client should be able to refuse to answer financial questions if he or she so desires.

Often the client's perception of his or her financial resources is at odds with the interviewer's perceptions. While the client's resources may appear to the interviewer to be adequate, the client may feel they are inadequate. For example, an air conditioner, which would provide relief for respiratory problems during the hot, humid summers, may be considered necessary by the clinician, but a luxury by the client, since it is too expensive to be purchased with a social security and/or pension check. Conversely, in some cases, the monthly income is so inadequate that the client is either continually incurring debts or not making necessary purchases (i.e., food, or fuel), but these clients may report that their income is adequate. A feeling of pride may prevent them from applying for public assistance.

Living Expenditures. Living expenditures demonstrate the manner in which the older adult uses personal resources to retain control over his or her life and environment. The financial demands made upon the individual and the ability to adequately meet these demands directly influences physical and mental well-being and quality of life.

Living expenditures are measured by 26 items related to housing, household operations, food, clothing, transportation, and recreation and leisure.

Reassessment

Through the 212 carefully selected items in the assessment instrument, the physical examination, and interaction with the client in the home setting, the Triage team is provided with the necessary information for developing a plan of care consonant with both the needs and values of the client. However, the assessment does not take place in a vacuum; the client's situation may change, and an intervention prescribed at one point in time may be inappropriate a few months (or weeks) hence. Thus, while an initial assessment is the crucial step in establishing a care plan, reassessment is also essential if that care plan is to remain up to date. The most appropriate interval between assessments seems to be six months.

To provide the team with an accurate picture of the client's changing status and needs, the reassessment does not have to include all items on the original assessment; background information has to be collected only once. For this reason, the Triage reassessment instrument is only about half the length of the original. The shorter length of the instrument means a corresponding shortening of the length of time needed for the reassessment interview. Although the time required for the reassessment is not long, the information gathered is invaluable in determining the impact of service and enabling appropriate changes in the plan of care to improve health status to the maximum possible extent.

Conclusion

Regardless of whether the goal of the plan of care is prevention, maintenance, or rehabilitation, a comprehensive data base obtained through the use of an assessment instrument, and translated into a problem-oriented record, is essential.

Only through a sensitive, thoroughly professional, multi-disciplinary assessment process, which takes into account the values as well as the needs of the client, can services be prescribed which are truly client-centered. Once the assessment is completed, a plan of care can be developed with the client and his or her family. The next step is to coordinate and monitor the necessary services to assure that they are meeting the client's needs, as identified through the assessment. This coordination and monitoring process is the subject of Chapter 5.

5

Service Coordination and Monitoring

NANCY RYAN, R.N., M.S.

The Triage assessment provides a single entry point for the delivery of medical and social services, but it is only the first step in assuring that care is delivered according to client need. After the comprehensive assessment of the older adult comes the difficult task of marshalling personal, family, and community resources to meet the identified needs, and insuring that the needs are indeed met on a continuing basis. The following three case studies illustrate the importance of this coordination and monitoring process.

Mrs. S.

Having recently experienced a mild myocardial infarction, Mrs. S., an 86-year-old widow, was discharged from an acute care hospital to her home under the care of her son, who took one week's vacation to be with her. In addition to her acute illness, Mrs. S. was wheelchair-bound with advanced rheumatoid osteoarthritis. Her son, who resided in her home, was addicted to alcohol and was on the verge of losing his job because of excessive absenteeism. Eight days after Mrs. S. had returned home, her granddaughter called Triage in desperation because her grandmother was still too weak to sit up in bed, much less transfer herself to her wheelchair; Mrs. S.'s son had to return to work after the weekend or lose his job; and the local visiting nurse association was unable to provide the necessary assistance. Who would help Mrs. S. take care of her basic needs?

Mr. A.

A local hospital home care coordinator contacted Triage for assistance with Mr. A., who had recently undergone his second mid-thigh amputation. Because Mr. A. no longer needed acute hospital care but refused nursing home placement, his physician discharged him to his mobile home under the care of his elderly wife. The hospital staff had assumed that Mr. A. would go to a nursing home, and therefore, had made no home preparation or evaluation of his wife's ability to provide home care for him. What did Mrs. A. need to know about caring for her husband? Were there architectural barriers in the home that would make it inaccessible for Mr. A.? Was Mrs. A. physically and emotionally able to accept her husband's disability and the resulting care that he might need?

Mrs. L.

Mrs. L. had referred herself to Triage "in case I ever need help." On initial assessment, she was found to be an active, healthy, 83-year-old woman who resided alone in her three room apartment. Her supportive daughters lived 30 to 50 miles away. Two months after self-referral, Mrs. L. fell and fractured her hip. While in the acute care hospital she was also treated for mild congestive heart failure. Upon discharge from the hospital, Mrs. L. was admitted to a skilled nursing facility. Three weeks after her admission to the nursing home, she was found to be both withdrawn and incontinent of urine. Because of her symptoms, she was diagnosed by the nursing staff and her physician as having irreversible organic brain syndrome. The physician advised her daughters that Mrs. L. would not be able to return to her apartment; therefore, the lease should be terminated. What was the cause of Mrs. L.'s deterioration? Were her symptoms due to the rapid changes in her environment or to her underlying physical problems? Was her condition reversible?

What do Mrs. S., Mr. A., and Mrs. L. have in common? Each one of them is an older adult who has multiple problems and needs two or more services. In addition, for a variety of reasons, each is unable to coordinate, on his or her own behalf, the services necessary to maintain independent living. Thus, each one is vulnerable to inappropriate, extended, or permanent institutionalization.

What transpired in the lives of Mrs. S., Mr. A., and Mrs. L. as a result of the Triage intervention? The initial assessment by the Triage professional team revealed that Mrs. S. was recovering slowly from her recent heart attack and needed continued assistance. Because her son had to return to work, he was unable to provide this assistance, and other arrangements had to be made. Several services were implemented by the Triage team immediately after the initial assessment. A home health aide was employed for eight hours per day, five days per week, providing personal care, preparing meals, and performing light housekeeping tasks, thus allowing the son to return to work and assuring client assistance and monitoring. A visiting nurse monitored the client's cardiac status; a physical therapist implemented a plan of progressive mobilization and transfer activities; and a physician agreed to make home visits, if necessary. Mrs. S. improved and became capable of transferring herself from bed to wheelchair to toilet. The home health aide's hours of service were gradually decreased to two hours per day and a telephone adapted to Mrs. S.'s special needs was installed. The visiting nurse's visits were decreased to once every other month, and the physical therapy was discontinued.

Mrs. S. remained a client for more than five years. Over time, her services were adjusted to meet her changing individual and family needs. During her final year of life, the home health aide was again present to assist for eight hours per day because Mrs. S. no longer had the strength to transfer or mobilize herself independently. Her son continued to work and controlled his alcohol problem. Because of appropriate, timely intervention, Mrs. S. was able to remain in her own home until 48 hours before her death.

Mr. A., upon hospital discharge following his second mid-thigh amputation, received a high level of services in order to stabilize both his medical condition and his home situation. Initially, a home health aide worked four hours per day to provide personal care to Mr. A. and to assist his elderly wife in transferring him from bed to wheelchair. The aide also provided some light housekeeping. A visiting nurse taught Mrs. A. how to care for her husband and how to meet her own personal needs. With physical therapy and special equipment, Mr. A. learned to transfer and mobilize himself in his small mobile home. As a result, the home health aide assistance was decreased to one hour each day for the personal care that Mrs. A. could not provide.

Mr. A. remained in his home for three years. After that time he had to enter a skilled nursing facility because his primary supporter, his wife, became terminally ill with cancer and was physically unable to continue to care for him. Despite their health problems, the emotional bond between Mr. and Mrs. A. remained strong. Through the efforts of the team to coordinate transportation, they were able to visit each other regularly. They were both extremely grateful that Triage devoted as much time and attention to their emotional needs as to their physical needs. When his wife died, Triage supported Mr. A. through his bereavement until the time of his own death six months later.

Our third example, Mrs. L., had been independent and very active before she was hospitalized for a fractured hip and subsequently placed in a nursing home. Based on the assessment, the Triage team believed that the diagnosis of irreversible organic brain syndrome was incorrect and that Mrs. L. was suffereing form severe situational depression. An attempt to have Mrs. L. moved from the nursing home to a re-habilitative hospital was aborted because that hospital confirmed the diagnosis of organic brain syndrome, although the hospital had only observed her for one day. The Triage team offered strong support to the family and convinced Mrs. L.'s daughters to transfer their mother to another nursing home in an adjacent town. Mrs. L. was unable to take part in the decision because of her depression. In the new environment, Mrs. L. received appropriate medical care, nursing care, physical therapy, and mental health counseling. After four months of intensive therapy, she was discharged from the nursing home to take up her life again functioning independently in the community.

The Long-Term Care Person

All elderly persons do not need comprehensive coordination and monitoring of health care services. However, many, like Mrs. S., Mr. A., and Mrs. L., do. They represent what has been referred to as "the long-term care person"* (Sherwood, 1975; Brody, 1977; Hickey, 1980)— individuals who have multiple stresses, such as functional disabilities and multiple physical and/or emotional handicaps. Such persons usu-ally need multiple health care services, often lack family or social

---

*Hickey (1980) devotes a section of his book *Health and Aging* to "the long-term-care person." He adopts the definition of Brody (1977): " . . . long-term care refers to one or more services provided on a sustained basis to enable individuals whose functional capacities are chronically impaired to be maintained at their maximum levels of health and well-being," and the term "long-term-care person" coined by Sherwood (1975) to refer to individuals at risk, as well as to those in need of or actually receiving services. He goes on to say: " . . . . In general, the long-term-care person is one who experiences limitations in daily activities and is regularly dependent on others to meet physical, medical, and/or functional needs."

supports, and generally have difficulty gaining access to or maneu-
vering through the health care system.

Coordination and monitoring of services should not be limited to
individuals receiving home care services, but should also be available to
individuals receiving institutional services. The basic goals should be
the same for clients in both settings. These goals are:

1. That the client function at his or her maximum level of
   independence, physically, emotionally, and socially;
2. That the client receive the appropriate level of services responsive to his or her needs at the right time; and
3. That the client receive services that are acceptable and of high
   quality.

Coordination of Service Delivery

While many forms of service coordination have been developed over
the years, home care programs which coordinate services between
the acute care hospital and the community are among those receiving
the most attention at the present time. Designed for a selected
population returning home from a hospital stay, the programs can be
either hospital or community based. Although they are a step in the right
direction, such programs have serious drawbacks. Generally, the only
individuals who participate are those whose physicians are aware of the
program and recognize the patient's need for it. In addition, the patient
must have insurance which reimburses for home services, or be able to
pay for the services out of pocket.

The assessment, coordination, and monitoring agency goes beyond
the concept of "extended" hospital care, where the goal is merely to
reduce the length of stay (and associated per diem cost) in an acute care
hospital, to a broader concept of coordination. From this perspective,
coordination is the process through which the professional team (composed of nurse-clinician and social service coordinator) implements a
service plan using the full spectrum of ambulatory, home health, and
institutional services.

The coordination effort is dynamic and not limited by time or
service type. With the traditional system, in contrast, client contact is
often terminated as soon as an acute problem is resolved. For instance,
when an individual is discharged from a hospital and enters a nursing

home, the physician who treated the acute episode may not continue to care for that person. If insufficient information is transferred from provider to provider, especially information that relates to the client's ability to function at home, the elderly person's stay in the nursing home may be unnecessarily long. And the longer older people remain in a nursing home, the more likely they are to lose the support they previously received from family, friends, and providers in the community—support they will certainly need if they are ever to return to their homes.

The amount of time and energy expended by the health professional in the coordination process depends upon:

1. The stability of the health status of the client;
2. The client's coping ability;
3. The client's ability to negotiate the delivery system;
4. The family support system;
5. Client acceptance and level of trust; and
6. The availability of appropriate service that is acceptable to the client and/or family.

For the well elderly, and for those who cope adequately and are able to negotiate the system, only minimal assistance in coordination may be necessary. For this population, the assessment process establishes a basis for quick intervention if health problems develop. Because there is baseline knowledge about the client's status, and an established relationship of trust between the professional and the client, timely intervention can be achieved. In contrast, for functionally disabled persons and those who require multiple home care services, the coordination efforts may be directed toward the continuous flow of direct service, thus preventing gaps in service provision.

Client Acceptance

In the implementation of a client-centered, coordinated care plan, a basic question is: How acceptable is the service to the individual? Many factors affect the older adult's acceptance of services. Fear, prejudices, values, level of understanding of the person's own health status, and attitudes toward health services and service providers must all be assessed to determine how the individual relates to the service delivery system. Often, the older adult fears the hospital as the place where one goes to die or where one has to accept charity because of limited financial resources. For many older adults, financial assistance is totally unacceptable; not only would they refuse charity for hospital expenses, they would choose to go without food rather than to accept "welfare."

To develop a viable plan of care, the coordinator of health services must not only understand the client's values, but accept them and work within the client's constraints. Keith-Lucas (1973) refers to this as "co-planning," a process which accepts the fact that while people are fallible, they generally are capable of managing their own affairs. The case of Miss C. illustrates this principle of co-planning.

Miss C.

Miss C., at 79 years of age, was still riding a two-wheeled bicycle. At the time of the initial assessment, she made it clearly known that she believed that women were smarter than men; all drugs were bad, and hospitals were not much better; and a proper diet supplemented with vitamins and minerals was essential to good health. Although Miss C. had not seen a physician or other health care professional in 30 years, she had significant medical and social problems, including hypertension, peripheral vascular disease, inadequate housing, and no personal support system.

It was essential to plan care in conjunction with Miss C.'s value system. A female physician outside the service area was obtained for Miss C., since the local female physician would accept her as a patient only if she were hospitalized for a complete medical evaluation. Miss C. was treated with Nicobid, a vitamin acceptable within her value system, yet therapeutic; she was provided with the personal support of the Triage team; and she was assisted with her housing problems. Five years later, Miss C. no longer rides her bicycle, but her hypertension is controlled and the circulation to her extremities has improved. This was accomplished because the coordinated care system was able to relieve her stress and support her within the confines of her beliefs.

Too often, health professionals determine appropriate services for the older person based on their own value systems. Kalish (1979) refers to these professionals as "geri-activists," faulting them for adhering to their own rigid standards of appropriate behavior. As the case of Miss

C. illustrates, older persons should be offered service options and be told about the assigned risks and benefits attached to each option. They should be the ones to decide what risks they choose to take, providing that complete information, options, limitations, and professional recommendations are offered. The ultimate decision is then theirs to make: Which option will best meet their needs and be consonant with their own values and goals?

In the "real world," the older adult does not always have the opportunity to make his or her own decisions. For example, the decision to place an elderly mother in a nursing home, often for the rest of her life, may be made by her family and physician. This decision may be based on the fear that she might fall, or the belief that caring for her has become too complicated.

An individual who has marked functional disability may be a prime candidate for 24-hour care because he or she may be unable to obtain immediate assistance if a problem arises. In this situation, the client may have to make an informed choice between entering a long-term care facility or remaining alone at home with intermittent assistance, risking the lack of immediate help in an emergency. Triage agrees with the point of view expressed by Flaconer, Altamura, and Behnke (1976) that " . . . to shelter the older person from all possible accidents is to shelter him from life." Conversely, involving the older person in the decision-making process makes that person feel adult, worthwhile, and competent.

Mrs. H.

Mrs. H., at 92 years of age, was a severely disabled woman who lived alone in elderly housing. Her sight had failed so that she could only see shapes, and, due to advanced osteoarthritis, she was unsteady when ambulating with her walker. Mrs. H. knew where everything was in her cluttered apartment as long as some well-meaning home care provider didn't clean up. It was not unusual for Mrs. H. to spend one night a month on the floor, having fallen after getting up in the middle of the night to go to the bathroom. She had experienced the alternative: being tied in a chair for three weeks in a skilled nursing facility because the staff feared she might fall. To Mrs. H., this arrangement was totally unacceptable.

As the result of the assessment and coordination process, Mrs. H. was able to return to her home. To maintain her at home, Triage coordinated the following services: a home health aide, one

hour a day, from 8 to 9 A.M., from a non-profit agency, and three
hours a day, from 5 to 8 P.M., from a proprietary agency; home
delivered meals every day at noon; and a monthly nursing visit to
pour her medications into individual envelopes. Even if Mrs. H.
had a problem and could not reach her phone or her neighbor did
not check on her, the coordinated care plan prevented her from
going more than several hours without assistance. With Triage's
help, she was able to enjoy independent living in her own home for
the next four years.

The value that the client places on the service will often be the
determining factor in the quantity, as well as the type, of service
prescribed. An individual who has maintained a spotless house all of
her life places a much greater value on homemaking service than does
the person whose home has always been extremely cluttered and
unkempt, and the former may therefore be willing to pay for additional
service hours out of her own pocket.

Trust Relationship

Much of the success in effective service coordination can be attributed
not only to the skill and expertise of the health care professional, but
also to the trusting relationship developed with the client. Having one
agency to call regardless of the nature of the problem develops trust
and familiarity and alleviates confusion. The client knows that help will
be available when it is needed.

Mrs. U.

At 2:30 A.M., Mrs. U. called for assistance because her
spouse, who had a severe mentation problem, was getting dressed
to go for a walk. The woman was distressed and confused about
how to handle the situation. Over the phone, the professional was
able to calm the woman and resolve the problem. Because there
was always someone to call in an anxious moment, the couple was
able to remain together at home, as they so strongly desired.

The establishment of the trust relationship with the client begins
with the initial assessment and builds with each client contact. The
ability of the professionals on the staff and the agency to respond to the
individual needs of the older adult in a non-judgmental fashion estab-

lishes a foundation for all future interactions. This foundation of mutual trust saves many hours of professional time in assisting the client as his or her needs change over time.

Mrs. M.

Mrs. M., an 85-year-old woman with multiple medical and social problems, resided with her single, working daughter in a squalid house. Although she required help with all the functions included in the Activities of Daily Living and Instrumental Activities of Daily Living indices, she initially refused the care of a medical doctor (she had seen a naturopathic physician in the past) and any other assistance. By respecting the values and fears of Mrs. M. and her daughter and developing a trusting relationship with them, and by supporting and working closely with direct service providers, the professional team facilitated Mrs. M.'s gradual acceptance of services. She allowed changes in her home to accommodate the home health aides and homemakers who worked with her between four to six hours a day, and agreed to a home visit by a medical doctor. With effective coordination and monitoring, Mrs. M. was able to die in her own home as she had fought so hard to do. Before she died, she had come to accept care that provided a safe environment and adequate health care.

Service Availability

"Have some wine, " the March Hare said in an encouraging tone.
Alice looked all around the table, but there was nothing on it but tea. "I don't see any wine," she remarked.
"There isn't any," said the March Hare.
"Then it wasn't very civil of you to offer it," said Alice angrily. (Carroll, 1946)

If care is to be truly client-centered, a broad array of services must first be a reality. If service options do not exist, then offering choices to the client will only prove meaningless. Service availability varies markedly from community to community, and even from one section to another within the same community. Those serivces less available to the elderly may include: financial management, chore work, companion services, evening hours for home health aides or homemakers, home-delivered meal service, and transportation. Service gaps are especially evident in rural areas. However, even if a service is available, it may not be accessible. Barriers to accessibility include: agency policies; census limitations; geographic restrictions; financial limitations; and physical or architectural structures which limit access (for example, a physician's office located on a second floor walk-up).

Coordination of services is a continuous process and, therefore, must be available on a 24-hour, daily basis for emergencies. It is not possible to confine all the problems of the frail or chronically disabled person to a 9 A.M. to 5 P.M. block of time, five days a week, the way traditional services have been available. It is equally inappropriate to use a hospital emergency room for non-emergency medical and social problems. Crises, as perceived by the client and/or family, may come on weekends or in the middle of the night. Although a crisis may seem minor to the health professional, it may appear major to the client or family. A health care delivery system that is unable to alleviate the fear of one's not receiving help at home when needed fosters inappropriate hospitalization, or permanent nursing home placement.

Choice of Provider

For the frail elderly person, the vast array of service providers, with their different policies, geographic regions, and types of services, makes service negotiation cumbersome, if not impossible. However, the coordinator of health care services who has a good knowledge of the community resources may assist clients in making informed choices from among the available services appropriate to their needs. In the selection of a service provider, the following questions should be considered:

1. Should the provider be an individual or a service agency?
2. If an agency is selected, should it be a single service or a multi-service agency?
3. Are the philosophy and policies of the direct care provider congruent with the client's value system?

When an individual plan of care requires several services, the coordination process might be eased if the services can be appropriately provided by a multi-service agency. Such an agency may provide better continuity of care. On the other hand, independent providers might be less restricted than would large agencies in accommodating themselves to the individual client's values.

Relations with Providers

The coordinator must develop a trusting, non-competitive relationship with the provider as well as with the client, and should be available as a resource for support and education. The home health aide who picks Mrs. H. up from the floor when she arrives in the morning must be reassured that risking an occasional fall while living independently at home is better for Mrs. H. than being tied in a chair in a nursing home. The relationship that the professional establishes with the service provider may enhance or hinder the coordination process. Personal contact and a working knowledge of a provider's capabilities, limitations, and procedures tend to help create a closer (and more timely) match of services to the older adult's needs.

The building of a relationship between the coordinating agency and the provider depends not only upon the professional team's knowledge of the provider, but also on the ability of team members to relate to the provider as one individual to another, thus offering an incentive for cooperation. Cooperation is also fostered when team members and providers mutually accept the client goals, when the coordinating staff can listen with empathy to the providers about job-related stresses, and when the coordinating agency arranges needed educational programs for the service providers. The establishment of strong inter-agency relationships not only assures better client care, but may also serve to encourage a provider to develop hitherto unavailable services.

Monitoring for Service Control

The coordinating agency enters its monitoring phase after the client's plan of care has been established. Monitoring for service control, both clinical and fiscal, is the process through which the professional team maintains regular contact with the older person, his or her family, and the providers to ensure that the services being delivered are congruent with the care plan and that they are meeting the individual's current needs both quantitatively and qualitatively. This function includes altering service plans as the older person's needs change.

Service monitoring should be related to the assessment and the subsequent goals established with the client. The frequency with which the team evaluates services will vary with the client's health status as it relates to goal attainment, the client and/or family's capabilities to evaluate the appropriateness of service, the type of service being provided, and the knowledge of the providers' usual quality of care.

As with the assessment and coordination process, clinical monitoring of services for quality and quantity requires that the health professional demonstrate diplomacy and tact, while being directive in guiding the service providers in the delivery of appropriate health care.

How much health care service should be prescribed is a question that relates to the functional level of the disabled person and his or her resources. At no time should personal resources be displaced; rather, help given by family, friends, and the immediate community should be supplemented. If undue stress on personal resources can be minimized for extended durations, often the very disabled individual can continue to be cared for at home. Sometimes all it takes is a few hours of relief a day, or even one or two weeks a year, for a family to be able to continue to care for the severely disabled.

To monitor services for quality and quantity requires the participation of both the client and the family. As in the care planning process, the client and family must be active participants in the monitoring of the services received. Clients residing alone with no family nearby are especially vulnerable and therefore need closer service monitoring than those who have strong family support. Families usually act as advocates for the client in obtaining satisfactory service and providing protection against abuse.

After a trust relationship with the client has been established, and the client has been assisted in both identifying needs and selecting services to meet those needs, the client should be able to help evaluate the services, describing which ones were satisfactory and which were unsatisfactory. Once a problem is identified, work with providers to effect change is necessary. If the client makes a financial contribution, even a minimal one, toward the payment of the services, he or she will generally place a higher value on the services, feel freer to criticize, and experience a greater sense of control.

Mechanisms to monitor the provider of service directly should include: on site observation; verbal and written reports; planned meetings with the provider; and a review of all bills that are related to client care. Personal observation may be accomplished at the time of a reassessment interview, through joint planning with the provider, or at unannounced visits to the client. These observations provide first-hand knowledge of the provider's performance (both skill and attitude). Written and verbal information from providers should describe the tasks performed and progress toward meeting established client-centered goals. A review of service bills provides an indication of adherence to or deviation from the prescribed plan of care. (Further details on the fiscal monitoring process can be found in Chapter 3.)

Different types of services present different problems in monitoring and effecting change. The difficulties may relate to the client's preferences or fears, the providers' policies, the providers' professional status, or state and federal regulations.

Home Health Aide/Homemaker Services

Home health aide and homemaker services are the most frequently delivered home care services. Although Medicare reimburses for only limited home health services, federal regulations do set minimal guidelines for their function and supervision. Thus, home health aides working with a Medicare-certified agency have had at least some training and are supervised. Because the Medicare regulations do not apply to non-certified agencies, the standards and supervision of these agencies vary markedly. Such agencies, therefore, usually require more careful monitoring than do certified agencies.

Monitoring problems are increased even more when non-agency personnel are utilized. Often, because of the cost or lack of manpower, families and/or individual elderly who desire home care advertise and hire help independent of agencies. Frequently, this independent person will have had no training and will not be supervised by qualified persons. When families or clients hire independent providers, they must be helped to understand how to evaluate the care provided. These independent service providers must be monitored closely for the continuity, safety, quality, and appropriateness of their services.

Visiting Nurse

Montoring of the visiting nurse service may be accomplished largely through written reports and individual conferences. The nurse's educational level, professional experience, and the quality of agency supervision will dictate the time needed to monitor this type of home care service. One area of concern is the identification of new client problems. Limited personal skill or experience, limited budget, and/or a system that is based on physician orders for care tend to foster tunnel vision; that is, new needs may not be identified, and thus, the care plan may not be adjusted to meet the client's changing needs.

Home-Delivered Meals

Home-delivered meals should be monitored on site, at both the place of preparation and at the client's home. In evaluating meals the professional must ask: Is there a therapeutic diet plan? Is there a cycle of meals for variety? Are the food handling, preparation, and packaging adequate? Do the meals look appetizing? When the meals are delivered, are hot foods hot and cold foods cold?

In addition to monitoring meal preparation and delivery, it is necessary to note what the client does with the meal. Does the client eat the meal at the time of delivery or does he or she reheat the meal later? Is it safe for the client to reheat the meal? Does the client actually eat the meal or does he or she stack the meals in the refrigerator? Does the client feed the meals to a pet? If the meals are not utilized properly, it is essential to determine why and to make an appropriate service change.

Mental Health Counseling

Whether short- or long-term, mental health counseling should be monitored not only through written reports, but also through individual goal-setting conferences. Goal-directed counseling is essential with the elderly because of the difficulty in changing long-established patterns of coping. Often it is a crisis or a change that interferes with these coping mechanisms. Therefore, counseling efforts should be directed toward assisting the older adult in developing skills to compensate for losses, to make decisions based on the present situation, and to cope with new life stresses. Short-term crisis intervention is usually a far more effective utilization of counseling for this age group than is long-term analysis.

One major difficulty with providing this service is that in the education and training of counselors, the needs of older adults have frequently been ignored. Another problem is the unwillingness of many older people to seek mental health services. Although it is generally believed that counseling is of more value when it is actively sought by the client, counselors must usually reach out in providing therapy for the elderly. With this age group, there continues to be a considerable stigma attached to mental health problems and mental health care.

Institutional Services

Acute hospitals and long-term care facilities require different monitoring practices than do home services. Services delivered in the home are delivered in a setting which maximizes the possibility for client control of the situation. In contrast, institutional services are delivered to a captive population and usually require elderly people to adjust and conform to policies and procedures which may conflict with their desires and life patterns.

To ensure that institutional care will be client-centered, the Triage team acts as an advocate for the client in an often alien environment. When a client is admitted to the hospital, the Triage team ensures that the hospital staff have the data essential to individualize care during the hospitalization as well as the information needed in planning for discharge at the earliest time consistent with high standards of care. They also assure that diagnosis, prognosis, and treatment options are communicated not only to the patient, but also to the patient's family or supporter.

Hospitalization is usually for only a short time period whereas placement in a nursing home may be for weeks, months, or even years. Thus, it is even more important that there be an advocate to monitor the quantity and quality of care received in a nursing home to ensure that the client does not become unnecessarily dependent.

When a client is admitted to a nursing home, client contact with the family support system is frequently restricted, thereby increasing the client's vulnerability. It is essential to monitor institutional care at different times during the day in order to evaluate whether there is consistency of care with changing shifts and staff. Frequent visits to an institution tend to stimulate staff interest in the older person, and thus have a positive effect on client care.

Reassessment

Just as assessment is the foundation of the coordinated system of care, formal client reassessment is the touchstone of the clinical monitoring process. While continuous monitoring must take place to ensure that the right services are being delivered at the right time and in the right quantity, a formal reassessment at fixed intervals (no greater than six months) is also necessary.

The reassessment is not only a review of the client's status, as described in Chapter 4, but also a review of services as they relate to client-centered goals. The central question to consider is how effective have the services been in meeting the goals of the individualized care plan. At the end of each reassessment, the assessor lists the services the client is receiving; examines the goal of each service (the restoration or maintenance of function, the prevention of deterioration, or the palliation of terminal illness); and then determines whether the goal has been met or unmet, and whether there is a need to continue to work toward existing goals or to establish new ones.

Impact on the Community

The coordination and monitoring of services by an independent agency which is not a direct service provider should not only have an effect on the quality and appropriateness of individual client care, but should also have an impact on service availability and service delivery in the community. As the older adult's health needs are identified, ways must be sought to meet these needs. The documentation of needed service will tend to stimulate the development of new types of services and to increase the availability of manpower, both formal (professional providers) and informal (friends and neighbors).

The stimulation of service development is achieved through cooperative relationships established with individual agencies and the community as a whole. One successful method that Triage utilizes to foster these relationships is the involvement of community representatives on an advisory committee. This committee, composed of a variety of professionals and agency administrators, provides a vehicle for continued inter-provider communication. By participating in the assessment, coordination, and monitoring agency's quality assurance program, and by reviewing its service policies, the committee members provide each other with valuable feedback and mutual encouragement for further service development.

Triage has also implemented educational and training programs for direct service providers. These programs have stimulated interest in the special needs of the older adult. Educational programs presented by the agency for visiting nurses, home health aides and homemakers, and nursing home staff afford these providers the opportunity to upgrade themselves professionally. By sharing the philosophy and purpose of holistic health care and presenting the knowledge and skills necessary to implement this approach, the educator has the opportunity to raise the standard of care delivered.

Conclusion

Triage has been described as the "system in-between," that is, the agency which provides an interface between the older adult and the community of providers. This system, which coordinates and monitors the multiple services and providers necessary to achieve client-centered care, has improved the comprehensiveness, continuity, and accessibility of services for the elderly.

While coordination and monitoring have had an impact at the community level, their value has been most fully realized at the individual level. The following excerpts from letters by two clients speak eloquently for the many other clients who have spontaneously expressed their gratitude for the Triage model:

> Thank you for the good help and service. It gave me inner strength to feel like a person. Each day has a new beginning, happy, independent, and sure that I was good taken care of.

Triage makes me feel as though for the first time I have a friend who knows me well, is always available, and has all the information I need to get help when I need it.

Robert Butler, the director of the National Institute on Aging, entitled his Pulitzer prize winning book on being old in America, "Why Survive?" He stated, "One tragedy of old age is not the fact that each of us must grow old and die, but that the process of doing so has been made unnecessarily and at times excruciatingly painful, humiliating, debilitating, and isolating . . . " (Butler, 1975).

Through its assessment, coordination and monitoring process, Triage enables its elderly clients to respond to the question "why survive?" in a positive manner. As one client so confidently wrote, "There are better days ahead for all of us, and the sun will also shine."

6
Project Evaluation

HELEN RAISZ, M.A.

Previous chapters have described the goals which Project Triage sets out to accomplish and the health delivery system designed and implemented to meet those goals. This chapter reports some of the preliminary findings of the evaluation research of Phase I of the Triage project, covering the three-year period 1976–1979 (Quinn, et al., 1979).

The purpose of the evaluation is to explore the hypotheses that coordinated care prescribed according to client need will, ideally, have two results: 1. The effectiveness of health services will be increased; and 2. expenditures for health services will be contained. Each of these hypotheses will be discussed in turn.

Effectiveness

The effectiveness of health services is defined in terms of functioning status. Coordinated services are regarded as effective if a client's functioning status is: improved, maintained, or, if neither of these outcomes is realistic, the rate and amount of deterioration is kept to a minimum. As Sherwood (1973) has stated:

> Change over time is not synonymous with impact. Impact is the difference between the state of affairs after the intervention and what it would have been without the intervention. From this point of view, 'no

change' in experimental subjects may in fact represent impact. An intervention program may be halting a debilitative process. If we looked at change measurements alone, it would seem as if nothing had happened. But if we had a sound basis to estimate that the condition would have deteriorated, and then found that at the second point of time it had not become worse, there would be reason to conclude that the intervention had positive impact. Indeed, very often the best we may expect to achieve is a slow-down in degenerative processes. *If we merely study the 'before and after' behavior of elderly persons being served by a rehabilitation program, we may be observing a downward pattern and assume failure when, in fact, without such a program deterioration would have been greater and have occurred at a faster rate.*

Three dimensions of overall functioning status, physical, mental, and social, are identified as the most important in determining an elderly individual's ability to remain independent. To measure these dimensions, three instruments—the Index of Independence in Activities of Daily Living, known as the ADL (Katz, et al., 1963), the Instrumental Activities of Daily Living, or IADL (Lawton & Brody, 1969), and the Mental Status Questionnaire, or MSQ (Kahn, et al., 1960)—are incorporated in the Triage assessment instrument. The ADL index assesses the level of independence in performing basic physical activities such as bathing, toileting, and feeding. The IADL measures more complex behaviors such as shopping, money management and housekeeping, which are instrumental in achieving general independence. The MSQ is a simple measure of cognitive ability which has been found to be a reliable indicator of change in reality perception.

Functioning status is measured twice: at the time of initial assessment, before the client receives coordinated care, and at the time of reassessment, after the client has received coordinated care for some period of time.

Client Description

Between the time Triage assessed its first client (March 1, 1974), and the end of enrollment for the first phase of the project (March 31, 1978), 2,128 clients were assessed. By the time ressessments began in September of 1978, the number of active clients had decreased to 1,404. The leading cause for this attrition was death (495 clients had died). This is not surprising since the average age for a Triage client at the time of assessment was 76 years of age. In addition to those who had died, 226 had withdrawn from the project (primarily because they had moved out of the region), and three were unavailable for reassessment at the scheduled time.

Sociodemographic Characteristics.   The Triage population included in this study (N = 2128) is, on the whole, slightly older than the elderly population of the nation. The median age of Triage clients is 76, compared to 73 for the elderly United States population. The percentage of the Triage population over 75 years of age is 57.5, compared to 27.0 percent for the nation's elderly.

There are some other noteworthy differences. Compared to the elderly United States population, the Triage population has a lower proportion of elderly males to females, a slightly higher proportion of widows, lower educational levels, and somewhat lower incomes. Thus, the group Triage serves is representative of the "frail elderly,"* consisting in large part of older, widowed women of limited educational attainment and less than adequate financial resources.

Functioning Status.   Initial functioning status scores reflect a relatively high degree of client independence in performing the seven basic activities of daily living (83.1 percent of the clients score six or better on the ADL scale of zero through seven), and of orientation to time and place (80 percent score eight or better on the MSQ scale of zero through ten). The IADL scores reflect the greater complexity of the instrumental activities of daily living. Whereas the majority of clients are independent in the functions measured by the ADL and MSQ, the majority of clients are relatively more dependent in IADL (only 34 percent score 6.5 or over on the IADL scale of zero through eight).

Findings: Changes in Functioning Status

Changes in functioning status were examined for the entire group of clients who remained active from the time of initial assessment to the time of final reassessment (N = 1404). The results showed Triage to be

---

*"By frailty is meant reduction of physical and emotional capacities and loss of a social-support system to the effect that the elderly individual becomes unable to maintain a household or household contacts without continuing assistance from others" (Federal Council on Aging, 1976).

more effective in improving or maintaining the scores of its clients on the MSQ and ADL than on the IADL. The proportion of clients who improved or maintained their scores was about 71 percent for both the MSQ and ADL, compared to 48 percent for the IADL (see Table 6–1).

The percentage of clients whose MSQ scores improved or were maintained can be attributed to several features of the Triage intervention. As Butler (1975) and Birren and Schaie (1977) have shown, many factors contribute to deteriorating intellectual functioning. Psychological factors (depression and stress-induced anxiety), nutritional deficiencies, social isolation, drug interactions, metabolic disorders, hospital-induced disorientations, and deteriorating overall physical functioning have all been implicated. Where warranted, Triage provides mental health counseling to treat depression and to alleviate anxiety. Nutritional deficiencies are corrected by well-balanced meal services. Social isolation is removed by friendly visiting. Careful monitoring of medications prevents or corrects adverse drug interactions. For specific metabolic intoxications, treatment by a team of internists and psychiatrists is provided.

The most difficult area in which to attain or maintain the maximum ability to function is the IADL. The smaller proportion of clients whose IADL scores improved or were maintained reflects not only the complexity of the individual tasks, but the fact that independence in these tasks depends on environmental factors beyond the control of the

TABLE 6–1. Changes in Functioning Status from Initial to Final Assessment

Scale	Improved/ Maintained		Declined		Total	
	No.	Percent	No.	Percent	No.*	Percent
MSQ	961	71.7	379	28.3	1,340	100.0
ADL	977	71.5	397	28.5	1,394	100.0
IADL	612	48.2	658	51.8	1,270	100.0

*N's are less than 1404 because of incomplete information on some clients.

client or the coordinating agency. For example, the ability to shop depends as much on the location of stores and the method of transportation available as on the physical and mental condition of the client.

While objective instruments such as the MSQ, ADL, and IADL are important outcome measures, subjective measures must also be considered. Between initial and final assessment, there was an increase of 10 percent (from 40 to 50 percent) in the proportion of clients who described their health as "good" or "excellent" and a concurrent decrease of 5 percent in the proportion who reported their health as poor. (The others described their health as "fair".) At the very least, the receipt of coordinated care appears to have improved client's perceptions of health. While empirical data on life satisfaction have yet to be examined, subjective information such as the outpouring of unsolicited testimonials by clients and their families suggests that, with a coordinated package of health and social services in place, the quality of clients' lives, as well as that of their families, has improved.

Expenditures

The second major goal of Project Triage is to contain expenditures for health services. The premise behind this goal is that expanding reimbursement through new service waivers to cover less expensive health care options, and providing assessment, coordination, and monitoring of all services through technical waivers, will effectively control costs without sacrificing the goal of client-centered, comprehensive care.

Consistent with the World Health Organization's (1980) definition of health as the equivalent of "physical, mental and social well-being," Triage defines the necessary spectrum of care as including a broad range of services designed to meet physical, mental, and social needs. This spectrum encompasses 24 types of medical and social services, which have been aggregated into five major groups: home health care, transportation, products, ambulatory care, and institutional services.

The basic questions posed by this aspect of the research are: what will it cost to provide client-centered care which integrates the multiple components of a coordinated medical and social service delivery system? And will the addition of new service waivers escalate the cost of care unreasonably?

To answer these questions, data were collected on the number of utilizers and the charge per client day for each of the 24 services during 1977 and 1978. Calendar year 1978 was the focus of the cost analysis because it was the time period most representative of the way in which an ongoing organization such as Triage would operate. Data for 1977 are presented for comparison purposes only (see Table 6–2).

In the discussion of expenditures which follows, the 24 services are presented by waiver type—new service waivers and technical waivers. The term "new service waivers" refers to the waivers which made possible reimbursement of services hitherto not covered. The term "technical waivers" refers to waivers of technicalities of currently-covered Medicare services such as "benefit period," "medical necessity," and "prior hospitalization." A fuller discussion of the waivers is presented in Chapter 3.

New Service Waivers

Utilization. The expansion of reimbursement to cover services such as homemaker, taxi, prescription drugs, optometry, and intermediate care facilities did not result in excessive or indiscriminate utilization of these services. Of the 12 newly waivered services, the only one utilized by over 50 percent of the clients was prescription drugs. Six services—non-prescription drugs, meals, chore, homemaker, taxi, and dentist—were used by 22 to 45 percent of the clients, while five services were utilized by 17 percent or fewer. Intermediate care facilities were utilized by only 2 percent of the clients.

Charges. The new service waivers did not result in significant additional costs. Further, the second year of the project (1978) showed a reduction in the charge per client day for six of these services, and an increase in only three. The most expensive of the new service waivers on a per client day basis was prescription drugs ($0.50 per client day) and meals ($0.49 a day). Charges for intermediate care facilities, companion, chore worker, counselor, and dentist were in the range of $0.10 to $0.20 per client day. Taxi, non-prescription drugs, optometry, and glasses were each under $0.04 per client day.

Technical Waivers

Utilization. In 1978 the most frequently used service in the technical waivers group was physician visits. Ninety-five percent of the clients received one or more visits per year. Fifty-one percent received diagnostic procedures. With the exception of these two services, no technically waivered service was used by more than 50 percent of the clients. Between 40 and 45 percent of the clients used visiting nurse, out-patient hospital, and podiatry services. The percentage of clients using home health aide and in-patient hospital services was approximately equal, 38 percent. Ambulance, equipment, and supplies were utilized by 20 to 25 percent and skilled nursing facilities by 18 percent. The least frequently utilized of the technical service waivers was therapy. Only 9 percent of the clients utilized this service.

Charges. In the second year, Triage contained costs in nine of the twelve categories of the technical waivers. The three services for which charges per client day were higher were out-patient hospital, physician services, and skilled nursing facilities. The charge per client day for therapist, diagnostics, and podiatry remained the same as it was in 1977. The charge per client day for visiting nurse, home health aide, equipment, supplies, and in-patient hospital services was lower.

Total Services

Utilization. Over the two-year period 1977–1978, only two services were consistently used by a large majority of the clients: physician services (a technical waiver) and prescription drugs (a new service waiver). None of the other services in the new service waiver category was used by over 50 percent of the clients in either 1977 or 1978. In the technical waiver category, two of the services, visiting nurse and diagnostics (in addition to physician services), were used by 50 to 53 percent of the clients in 1977. In 1978, only one service, diagnostics, was used by more than half the client group.

Charges. Average charges for all 24 types of service per client day were $11.45 in 1977 and $11.31 in 1978. When services for 1978 were analyzed according to typical usage profiles, and charges were excluded

TABLE 6-2. Percent of Clients Utilizing Services and Charge Per Client Day

Service Group	1977		1978	
	Percent of Clients Utilizing	Charge Per Client Day	Percent of Clients Utilizing	Charge Per Client Day
I. Home Health Services				
Technical Waivers:				
Visiting Nurse	53	.40	45	.31
Home Health Aide	41	1.03	38	.90
Therapist	11	.08	9	.08
Sub-total		1.51		1.29
New Service Waivers:				
Homemaker	24	.40	22	.31
Chore*	27	.14	23	.14
Companion*	6	.18	6	.15
Sub-total		.72		.72
II. Transportation				
Technical Waiver:				
Ambulance/Chair car	27	.10	25	.09
New Service Waiver:				
Taxi	28	.02	24	.02
III. Products				
Technical Waivers:				
Equipment	25	.18	20	.16
Supplies	31	.05	24	.03
Sub-total		.23		.19

New Service Waivers:				
Prescription Drugs	99	.45	91	.50
Meals*	36	.58	29	.49
Non-prescription Drugs	45	.03	32	.02
Glasses/Hearing Aid	17	.04	23	.05
Sub-total		1.10		1.06

IV. Ambulatory

Technical Waivers:				
Physician	95	.86	95	1.01
Diagnostic	50	.09	51	.09
Podiatrist	41	.06	40	.06
Outpatient Hospital	42	.22	42	.28
Sub-total		1.24		1.45
New Service Waivers:				
Optometry/Audiology	9	.01	9	.01
Dentist	22	.10	22	.15
Counselor*	10	.11	6	.02
Sub-total		.21		.17

V. Institutional Services

Technical Waivers:				
Hospital	39	3.69	37	3.55
Skilled Nursing Facility	17	2.43	18	2.76
Sub-total		6.12		6.31
New Service Waiver:				
Intermediate Care Facility	2	.20	2	.13
Sub-total		.20		.13
TOTAL FIVE SERVICE GROUPS				
Technical Waivers		9.20		9.33
New Service Waivers		2.25		1.98
Total		11.45		11.31

* = Triage negotiated rate.

for those very ill clients who remained in the program for less than a year, the charges per client day dropped to $9.77. Apparently, then, the very ill group had much higher per-client-day charges, which can be attributed to the repeated hospitalizations that they required.

Charges for many services were only pennies a day. Per-client-day charges were $0.10 or less for each of the following services: dentist, glasses, non-prescription drugs, taxi, ambulance, diagnostics, therapy, podiatry, supplies, and optometry/audiology. The only services incurring charges of a dollar a day or more in both 1977 and 1978 were hospital and skilled nursing facility. In 1977, the charges per client day for home health aide service were also over $1.00; and in 1978, the charges for physician service exceeded $1.00. The rest of the services ranged from $0.11 to $0.58 per client day in 1977, and from $0.13 to $0.50 in 1978, for the newly waivered services; and from $0.18 to $0.86 in 1977, and from $0.16 to $0.90 in 1978, for the technically waivered services.

An examination of the percentage distribution of the 24 service types suggests that Triage has effected a shift away from the emphasis on hospitals and physicians prevalent in the current system toward comprehensive home health care. Percentage distributions of personal health care expenditures for the U.S. population 65 and over (Fisher, 1980) have been compared to these Triage distributions. In 1978, the distribution of expenditures for hospital care was 12 percent lower for Triage clients than for the U.S. elderly as a whole (31 percent compared to 43 percent); and for physician services, 9 percent compared to 18 percent.

There was considerable risk in developing the Triage project with its broad set of waivers, its easy access to care, and its signal departure from what we know as the traditional system. However, the evaluation demonstrated that care was rendered at a total cost not significantly greater than the cost of the limited set of services available within the traditional Medicare system. Further, the charge per client day for new service waivers was not only contained, but was actually reduced by 12 percent at a time when unit costs were rising.

The experience of Triage gives hope that the elderly can receive client-centered care, care that is not only humane from the point of view of the elderly and their families, but efficient from the point of view of the not yet elderly whose contributions to the Medicare Trust Funds make such a system of care a reality.

7

Implementation Potential

HELEN RAISZ, M.A. AND JOSEPH HODGSON, M.S.W.

The Triage model of client-centered care represents one solution to the problem of care of the frail elderly. It is an approach that has succeeded in containing the costs of care without sacrificing quality. To date, this model has been tested only in the seven-town Central Connecticut region. The findings of the study warrant the continued testing on a nationwide basis of a comprehensive assessment, coordination, and monitoring system with reimbursement oversight. If the process is to be transferable to other parts of the country, issues such as the level of staff expertise, geographical and cultural considerations, regional availability of service, and the interaction of potentially similar client population groups must be addressed. However, there do not seem to be any insurmountable technical obstacles standing in the way of replicating the model with local variations. Recent administrative and legislative initiatives embody many of the concepts and features of the Triage model.

Administrative Initiatives

A major administrative response has been to mount a national long-term care channeling demonstration (see Chapter 1 for a definition of channeling). This program "is intended to meet a current need of the government by producing information that will lead to administrative and legislative initiatives for developing a more effective long-term care system" (U.S. DHEW, 1980).

The Department of Health and Human Services has established the following four objectives for the national program:

1. To stimulate improvements at the state and community level in the organization and orientation of the long-term care delivery system, the relationships between service providers, and the way long-term care resources are distributed and controlled.
2. To demonstrate and measure the effectiveness of various channeling approaches for managing long-term care resources within a community on behalf of individual clients.
3. To collect comparable information on the impact of channeling on costs, services utilization, and client outcomes to assist the Department, states, and communities in the development of more humane and effective long-term care policies.
4. To develop a greater understanding of the population which needs and uses long-term care.

On September 29, 1980, awards were granted to 12 states to establish statewide channeling agencies. These channeling agencies will build on demonstration projects such as Triage and other model prototypes such as: Monroe Community Long-Term Care, Wisconsin Coordinated Care for the Elderly, Georgia Alternative Health Services, Washington Community-Based Care for the Functionally Disabled, Mount Zion Long-Term Care for the Frail Elderly, Minnesota Health Seniors Center, and New York Long-Term Health Care.

Legislative Initiatives

During the past few years, several major pieces of legislation which proposed solutions to the current institutional bias of the health system have been introduced into Congress. One, the Medicaid Community Care Act of 1980 (H.R. 6194), sponsored by Representatives Claude Pepper and Henry Waxman, called for comprehensive assessments and community-based services to Medicaid institutionally-eligible individuals. Under the provisions of this bill, a state which has a community care plan would be eligible for up to a 90 percent federal share with respect to comprehensive assessments and nine community-based services such as nursing, home health aide, medical supplies (equipment and appliances), therapy, audiology, adult day health, respite care, homemaker and nutritional counseling. Administration would be through the state Medicaid agency, whose responsibility it would be to coordinate services with Titles XVIII and XX.

A second important piece of legislation, the Medicare Long Term Care Act of 1979 (H.R. 58, introduced by Representative Barber Conable), would amend Title XVIII to establish a long-term care Trust Fund financed by premiums from enrollees and, if necessary, federal appropriations. The bill proposed the creation of state long-term care centers as part of a new administrative structure for the organization and delivery of services, for which the federal government would pay a 90 percent share. Nursing home services as well as home health services would be covered, but not physicians and hospitals.

A third significant bill, which incorporated many features of the client-centered model, was S.2809, "Non-Institutional Long-Term Care Services for the Elderly and Disabled" (known as Title XXI of the Social Security Act). Introduced by Senator Robert Packwood, this bill would amend the Social Security Act to provide for a program of comprehensive, community-based, non-institutional long-term care services.

Title XXI would coordinate home health and in-home services for the elderly and disabled by removing them from Titles XVIII, XIX, and XX and translating them into homemaker/home health aide adult day services and respite services under a new Title. In addition, the assessment function would be incorporated through the establishment of Preadmission Screening and Assessment Teams (PAT's). Only those services recommended in a PAT's plan of care would be reimbursed. All the technical waivers to home health care incorporated in the Triage model are included. However, Title XXI would perpetuate the dichotomy between institutional and non-institutional care, because nursing home care would not be covered. It also would continue the distinction between acute and chronic illness, since utilization of home health as a way of recuperating from an acute episode would remain covered under Title XVIII, rather than being covered under the new Title XXI. Several essential services would not be included under Title XXI, such as meals-on-wheels, drugs, transportation, respiratory therapy, chore services, and companion care.

While these three bills have proposed rather ambitious changes in the present legislation, thus far, progress has been made in smaller increments. For example, the Omnibus Reconciliation Act of 1980 (P.L. 96–499) authorized several changes in the Medicare program, including technical waivers that:

1. Allow unlimited home health care visits;
2. Remove the requirement for three days of hospitalization prior to home health services under Part A of Medicare;
3. Delete the $60 deductible for Part B home health benefits;
4. Eliminate state licensing requirements for home health agencies;
5. Create a regional fiscal intermediary system.

Agenda for the Eighties

While administrative and legislative initiatives give reason for optimism, other social currents give equally persuasive reasons for pessimism. In the words of the director of the National Institute of Aging, Robert Butler, "we are confronted by a politics of austerity . . . marked by fear and retrenchment, increasing conservatism and possible intellectual and scientific stagnation" (Butler, 1980). At this time, according to Robert Binstock, Director of Brandeis University's Program in Economics of Aging, the United States is facing "a painful dilemma . . . whether to retrench our collective responsibilities toward the elderly or increase our efforts to alleviate the problems of older persons at the cost of other national goals" (Binstock, 1980).

How much of the nation's resources will be devoted to solving the problem of the care of the frail eldery? Perhaps the most valuable ally the elderly have in the clash between interest groups is that they are us. When we talk of the aged in the abstract, we are talking about our future selves. If we wish to have the advantages of a humane, client-centered approach to long-term care in our own old age, we must build the foundation now.

Bibliography

Amster, L.E., and Krauss, H.H. The Relationship between Life- Crises and Mental Deterioration in Old Age. *International Journal on Aging and Human Development 5*: 51–55, 1974.

Binstock, R. What Should Our Goals Be for the Eighties and Beyond? In *Aging: Agenda for the Eighties*. National Journal Conference Proceedings. Washington, D.C.: The Government Research Corporation, 1980.

Birren, J.E., and Schaie, K.W. *The Psychology of Aging*. New York: Van Nostrand Reinhold, 1977.

Blenkner, M. The Normal Dependencies of Aging. In *The Dependencies of Old People*, R. Kalish (ed.). Ann Arbor: Institute of Gerontology, 1969.

Bloom, S., Connecticut Commission on Aging. Letter to Governor Meskill, 15 October 1971.

Brody, E.M. Congregate Care Facilities and Mental Health of the Elderly. *Aging and Human Development 1*:279–321, 1970.

Brody, E.M. *Long-Term Care of Older People: A Practical Guide*. New York: Human Sciences Press, 1977.

Brotman, H.B. Every Ninth American. *Developments in Aging*. Special Committee on Aging, U.S. Senate, 1978.

Butler, R. The Triumph of Survivorship: Opportunities for Society. In *Aging: Agenda for the Eighties*. National Journal Conference Proceedings. Washington, D.C.: The Government Research Corporation, 1980.

Butler, R. *Why Survive? Being Old in America*. New York: Harper and Row, 1975.

Caroll, L. *Alice's Adventures in Wonderland and Through the Looking Glass*. Cleveland: The World Publishing Co., 1946 (1862).

Congressional Budget Office, Congress of the United States. *Long-Term Care for the Elderly and Disabled*. Washington, D.C.: U.S. Government Printing Office, 1977.

Cousins, N. *Anatomy of an Illness as Perceived by the Patient*. New York: Norton, 1979.

Doherty, N., Segal, J., and Hicks, B. Alternatives to Institutionalization for the Aged: Viability and Cost Effectiveness. *Aged Care and Services Review 1*:1–16, 1978.

Falconer, M., Altamura, M.V., and Behnke, H.D. *Aging Patients: A Guide for Their Care*. New York: Springer Publishing Co., 1976.

Federal Council on Aging. *Public Policy and the Frail Elderly*. DHEW Publication No. (OHDS) 79–20959, December, 1978.

Fisher, C. Differences by Age Groups in Health Care Spending. *Health Care Financing Review 1*:65–90, Spring 1980.

Fuchs, V. *Essays in Economics of Health and Medical Care*. New York: Columbia University Press, 1972.

Galblum, T.W. Research on Demonstrations in Health Care Financing, 1978–

1979. HCFA Publication No. 03044. Baltimore: U.S. Department of Health and Human Services, Health Care Financing Administration, 1980.

General Accounting Office, Comptroller General of the U.S. *Home Health— The Need for a National Policy to Better Provide for the Elderly.* Washington, D.C., (HRD 78–19), December 30, 1977.

Glick, P. A Demographic Look at American Families. *Journal of Marriage and Family 37*:15–26, 1975.

Hickey, T. *Health and Aging.* Monterey, Calif: Brooks/Cole Publishing Co., 1980.

Holmes, T.H., and Masuda, M. Life Change and Illness Susceptibility. Symposium of the American Association for the Advancement of Science, Chicago, December 1970.

H.R. 58. *Medicare Long-Term Care Act of 1979.* U.S. Congress, Washington, D.C.

H.R. 6194. *Medicaid Community Care Act of 1980.* U.S. Congress, Washington, D.C.

Kahn, R.L., Goldfarb, A.I., Pollack M., and Gerber, I.E. The Relationship of Mental and Physical Status in Institutionalized Aged Persons. *American Journal of Psychiatry 117*:120–124, 1960.

Kalish, R. The New Aging and the Failure Model: A Polemic. *The Gerontologist 19*:398–402, 1979.

Kamerman, S. Community Services for the Aged: The View from Eight Countries. *The Gerontologist 16*:529–537, 1976.

Katz, S., and Akpom, C. A Measure of Primary Sociobiological Function. *International Journal of Health Services 6*:493–508, 1976.

Katz, S., Ford, A.B., Moskowitz, R.W., Jackson, B., and Jaffe, M. Studies of Illness in the Aged: The Index of ADL, A Standardized Measure of Biological and Psychosocial Function. *Journal of the American Medical Association* 185:914–919, 1963.

Keith-Lucas, A. Philosophies of Public Social Services. *Public Welfare 31*:21–24, Winter 1973.

Lawton, M.P. The Functional Assessment of Elderly People. *Journal of the American Geriatrics Society 19*:465–481, 1971.

Lawton, M.P., and Brody, E.M. Assessment of Older People: Self-Maintaining and Instrumental Activities of Daily Living. *The Gerontologist 9*:179–186, 1969.

Lawson, I.R. A Taxonomy of Geriatric Care Using the Problem-oriented Record System. In *The Language of Geriatric Care: Implications for Professional Review.* I.R. Lawson and S.R. Ingman (eds.). Connecticut Health Services Research Series, No. 6:24–26, 1975.

Leopold, E., and Schein, L. Missing Links in the Human Services Non-system. *Medical Care 13*:595–606, 1975.

Litman, T. Health Care and the Family: A Three Generational Analysis. *Medical Care 9*:67–81, 1971.

Lowenthal, M.F. Antecedents of Isolation and Mental Illness in Old Age. *Archives of General Psychiatry 12*:245–254, 1965.

National Academy of Sciences. A Policy Statement: The Elderly and Functional Dependency. Washington, D.C.: Institute of Medicine, National Academy, June 1977.

Neugarten, B.; Havighurst, R.; and Tobin, S. The Measurement of Life Satisfaction. *Journal of Gerontology 16*:134–143, 1961.

Osler, W. *Aequanimitas*. New York: McGraw-Hill, 1906.

P.L. 92–603. *The Social Security Amendments of 1972*. U.S. Congress, Washington, D.C.

P.L. 96–499. *Omnibus Reconciliation Act of 1980*. U.S. Congress, Washington, D.C.

Quinn, J., Hicks, B., Raisz, H., and Segal, J., (eds.). Triage: Coordinated Delivery of Services to the Elderly. Final Report. Plainville, CT: Triage, Inc., December 1979.

Quinn, J.L., and Ryan, N.E: Assessment of the Older Adult: A 'Holistic' Approach. *Journal of Gerontological Nursing* 5:13–18, March, April 1979.

S. 2809. *Non-Institutional Long-Term Care Services for the Elderly and Disabled*. U.S. Congress, Washington, D.C.

Shanas, E., et al: *Old People in Three Industrial Societies*. New York: Atherton Press, 1968.

Sherwood, S: The Impact of Home Care Service Programs. Prepared for Gerontological Society Conference, San Francisco, California, June 28–29, 1973.

Sherwood, S. (ed.). *Long-term Care: A Handbook for Researchers, Planners, and Providers*. New York: Spectrum Publications, 1975.

Taber, M. Wicked Problems. *The Gerontologist* 20:247–248, 1980.

Terris, M., Cornely, P.B., Daniels, H.C., and Kerr, L.E. One Case for a National Health Service. *American Journal of Public Health* 67:1183–1185, 1977.

U.S. Department of Health, Education, and Welfare. *Health Insurance Administrative Costs*, SSA–76–11856. Washington, D.C.: U.S. Government Printing Office, 1976.

U.S. Department of Health, Education, and Welfare. *Your Medicare Handbook*, SSA–79–10050. Washington, D.C: U.S. Government Printing Office, 1979.

U.S. Department of Health, Education, and Welfare, Office of the Assistant Secretary for Planning and Evaluation, Division of Contract and Grant Operations. Request for Proposal, RFP-74-80-HEW-05, April 25, 1980.

Weed, L.L. *Medical Records, Medical Evaluation, and Patient Care*. Cleveland: Case Western Reserve University Press, 1971.

Weiler, P. *Adult Day Care: Community Work with the Elderly*. New York: Springer, 1978.

Williams, T.F. Appropriate Placement of the Chronically Ill and Aged: A Successful Approach by Evaluation. *Journal of the American Medical Association 226*:1332–1335, 1973.

World Health Organization. Constitution of the World Health Organization. In *Basic Documents*, 30th ed. Geneva, 1980.

Index

Index

Acceptance of services, 87–90
Activities of Daily Living (ADL), 78–79, 102, 103, 104, 105
Administrative initiatives, 111–112
Administrative staff, Triage, 22–23
Age, assessment of, 66–68
Alternative concept of long-term care, 4–5
Ambulance services, 39, 41, 59–60, 107, 108, 110
Ambulatory services, 39, 41, 47–52, 106, 107, 109, 110
Ancillary medical services, 39, 41, 52–53
Assessment
  client description, 102–103
  defined, 64
  holistic approach to, 64–81
  in Triage budget, 28, 30
Assessment instrument, 64–66, 80–81, 82–84
  dental information, 74–75
  economic items, 79
  environmental assessment, 69
  family support, 70–71
  functioning status (ADL/IADL), 78–79
  living arrangements, 69–70
  medical treatment, 72–73

  medications, 73–74
  nutrition, 75
  physical examination, 74
  physical health and medical items, 71–74
  psychological items, 76–78
  reassessment, 80
  sensory impairment, 75–76
  social functioning, 70
  social items, 66–71
Audiology, 41, 47, 50–51, 109, 110

Caseworkers, role tension with nurse-clinicians, 19–21
Central Connecticut Planning Region, 15
Chaircar services, 39, 41, 59–60, 107, 108, 110
Channeling agency concepts, 4, 111–112
Choreworkers, 39, 41, 54–55, 95–96, 108
Claims processing, 22–23, 61–62, 63
  and Triage budget, 28, 29, 30
Client
  acceptance of services, 87–80
  assessment of, see Assessment instrument
  description of, 102–103